YAEL DREZNIK

And the night has yet to come

Yael Dreznik

And the night has yet to come

Edited by: Melanie Shapiro

As a member of the medical profession, I solemnly pledge to dedicate my life to the service of humanity. The health and well-being of my patient will be my first consideration (The doctor's oath, Declaration of Geneva)

This book is dedicated with love and longing to Ronen, David, and Daphna.

May your souls rest in peace.

Table of Contents

5 a.m.

"Reminder to everyone, morning round at 6, lots of new patients", flashes a message from Puta on the residents' WhatsApp group.

It's dawn, and the first rays of sunlight illuminate the corner of the bedroom. I roll over, but the alarm clock on my phone keeps ringing. I glance at Gadi in a deep sleep next to me, turn off the alarm and get out of bed. Another long day ahead of me, I think to myself as I get dressed, the reflection of my green uniform visible in the large mirror opposite me.

Over the past two years, it has become a regular ritual to set my alarm for 5 a.m., a ridiculous hour to get up, let alone remain sane until the end of my workday at 9 p.m., or worse still, until the following morning on a 26-hour on-call shift such as today.

I don't remember a morning when I saw my girls awake. They are always asleep at this hour; disheveled hair, their bodies warm and sweet-smelling, Nitzan with the pillow over her head, as always, from when she was a baby, and Tamar with the door closed in complete darkness. I go to the living room, turn on the computer and inspect the list of new patients admitted to the ward. I brace myself for another day of war. On-call shifts like today provoke a sense of fear, a nervous stomach and agitation that never abate. Despite the experience and confidence I've gained since the start of my residency, the fear of the unknown constantly hovers over me and sometimes I feel it's all too much.

A week ago, when I inserted a chest tube, all by myself, into a young man who had been injured in a car accident, I felt alone for the first time, wondering what would happen if I were to accidentally penetrate his heart or make some other error... dear God! There would be no one to hold my hand, which at times is what I need most.

8

I park in the hospital parking lot. It's 5:45 a.m. and as the sun climbs above the cardiology building, I feel it's welcome warmth. Luckily, it's still summer and warm, because I am at my worst when I am both cold and tired. When I was young, I and my friend Inbal, whom I have known since the age of three, once tried to establish what the worst combination of unpleasant feelings is at any given time. We came to the conclusion that being hungry, having a headache, feeling cold and needing to pee, had to be the worst. But back then, I didn't yet know what it was like to work in the ER as the attending surgeon with forty patients waiting to devour me like a pack of wolves, or to stand cowering in a corner of the OR while a senior surgeon barks at me.

I hurry to the ward round. The night shift nurses are filling out the end-of-shift report and preparing for handover. We residents, the 'blue side' or 'Puta's side' as we call it, prepare for our morning round. Puta is like my big brother here. Even though he began his residency only a year ago, hierarchy on the surgical ward is similar to that of the military, or in Puta's words (he served in an elite unit in the army where he became boorish and brought some of his crassness to the ward): "It's enough for someone to be in residency a day longer than you for them to be considered your senior." And this is how it is with Puta, Imrish and myself; Puta is the senior resident, Imrish the less senior resident, and I, the newest resident, who does all the dirty work and keeps out of everyone's way.

Puta is a master of patient management. Some call him 'the magician' because he knows exactly when a surgical patient ceases to be a surgical patient and becomes an internal medicine patient.

"Did you see that Mrs Berkowitz passed a stool, Dreznik?" Puta quips. "It means she has no bowel obstruction. It's time to introduce her to the internal ward because she has pneumonia."

Imrish, who began his residency six months after Puta, is a real charmer, aided by his long forelock, contemplative look and great sense of humor. It was into this 'gutter' that I was thrown, and every day the three of us try to survive the morning round and finish it by 8 a.m. so we can get to the OR.

"Are you doing a lumpectomy with Dr Kleiman today, Dreznik?" Imrish asks me, after we finish going over the 'iron'—the tattered binder that lists the day's tasks, such as blood tests, scheduled colonoscopies, angiographies and CTs for the patients on the ward. Dr Kleiman is one of the veteran doctors in the department; an excellent yet very intimidating surgeon in the OR. Imrish always turns pale when he recalls how two weeks earlier he had failed to wake up in time for surgery with Kleiman, which meant only one thing: He had violated Kleiman's law of punctuality; a sin for which the only atonement is death.

Luckily for Imrish, Puta was willing to cover for him and prepare for surgery in the OR, so that when Imrish arrived—breathless, goggle-eyed, a pillow crease still on his face—he could take over. Just listening to this story, which in the last two weeks has been told over and over on various resident forums, including Puta's accurate and nonchalant account of how quickly Imrish scrubbed in, was enough to stress me out for today's surgery, and I hope it will end quickly. As residents, we are eager to get to surgery, but there are times when I would rather sit in the ward than suffer in the OR, and today is one of those times.

Since the early days of medical school, I knew I wanted to specialize in general surgery. My first encounter with a cadaver was during a visit to the morgue as part of my practical anatomy studies at Tel Aviv University's Faculty of Medicine. As I, Zehavit—my best friend in medical school—and a hundred other students made our way down to the morgue, we were struck by the pungent smell of formalin. There we stood, clad in scrubs, equipped with a scalpel and tweezers, staring in horror at dozens of cadavers on iron bunks, each wrapped in a blue towel. I can only describe it as the most hallucinatory and stressful experience I have ever had. Shortly before this chilling encounter, we had trepidly gathered in the university lobby with our anatomy books and listened to the department secretary explain the code of conduct in the dissection room. At one point I remember turning to look at Zehavit and saw her gazing back at me, our eyes watery with fear and apprehension.

In our cadaver dissection classes, we first learned about the back muscles and only later we were exposed to the head of the cadaver, supposedly in an attempt to lessen the initial shock. Each group of six students was assigned a dissection instructor, whom the students stood around, and when he made the first incision and exposed the *latissimus dorsi* and the *trapezius*, there was a deafeningly silence in the room.

Already back then I knew I wanted to hold a scalpel. One always hears of students who faint at their first dissection or drop out of medical school soon after, but in our class no one fainted or quit; we all stuck it out and survived. Even when we peeled off the skin of a cadaver and I lost my appetite until the following morning, I knew I would be a surgeon. But the exact field of surgery I would end up in—cardiothoracic, general or neurosurgery—I didn't yet know.

I scraped through the dissection classes before moving on to my clinical years, only to realize that I am not cut out for internal medicine. The hodgepodge of internal diseases—heart failure, kidney failure, urosepsis infections—and elderly patients who deteriorate before your eyes, while the internist balances them with medications and fluids, was more than I could bear. So, in truth, it was only by virtue of the occasions I was awarded the opportunity to sew incisions, remove ports and actively participate in appendectomies, that I got through my sixth year of medical school. At that stage Puta was still an intern and Imrish hadn't yet arrived on the scene, yet I had already secured my future in the surgical department without knowing how much blood, sweat and tears were ahead of me.

It's 5:55 a.m. We stand like soldiers in formation in front of room 1 in the long corridor of the surgical ward. With us are three apprehensive interns, waiting for Puta to bark at them. The rooms farthest from the nurses' station are naturally occupied by patients whose condition is stable. On each side, the blue and the red, there are about thirty patients to examine and decide how to proceed with treatment for each one: who to discharge, who to send for further tests, who for post-operative assessment, and so forth. The most recent resident to join the hospital, namely me, is in charge of documenting all this on the laptop. In years to come, when I am asked where I learned to touch type, I will reply, without hesitation—in general surgery.

"Shit," Puta mutters quietly, as we stand next to Aaron's bed. A week earlier, Aaron had undergone a total gastrectomy due to a large tumor, and he was about to be discharged. His abdominal drainage looked good and today we had hoped to remove one of the drains. Yesterday his wife, Leah, visited and together we teased Aaron about not eating a donut in case it got stuck in his throat. This silly joke put a smile on Aaron's face, and in recent days he has begun to touch my heart. It's amazing how quickly we form a bond with a patient, as they lie there, their body spread out on the bed, their soul screaming through anxious eyes. Just as Aaron's soul is screaming at us now as Puta picks up the drain for us all to see, and says in a somber voice: "The drain looks pancreatic, he has a pancreatic leak...inform Dr Vasser. Start Aaron on Tazocin right away and move him closer to the nurses' station as quickly as possible."

6 a.m.

Imrish, Puta and I are looking at Aaron's cloudy drainage, when Leah enters the room with a smile on her face and a bag of candy for the staff. She slowly gazes at the three of us in turn.

"I'm sorry," Puta says to Leah, with as much empathy as he can muster at this early hour of the morning and with 20 more patients to examine, "but the fluid in the drain doesn't look good, so we need to move Aaron to a room close to the nurses' station, give him antibiotics and see what happens. He must fast from now on, of course." Leah places the bag of candy aside and looks at me with questioning eyes. I leave the room with her for a minute before Puta has time to reprimand me for abandoning the round. It's the most frustrating feeling, I think to myself, when something goes wrong at the last minute—after months of chemotherapy, radiation and major surgery—that shatters the excited anticipation of going home. Leah wipes a tear from the corner of her eye and I have a dry feeling in my mouth as I try to lift the fog around Puta's explanation. As Leah eventually gathers herself together and tells me that she hopes, with God's help, that everything will be okay, the nurses arrive and move Aaron closer to their station.

I follow Aaron and Leah with my eyes and see her look anxiously at her husband with puffy eyes from crying. I recall being with them just two weeks ago at the pre-op clinic, where Aaron did tests, gave his medical history and received information about the surgery. The pre-op clinic is a bit like an assembly line that begins with the nurse, continues with the intern and ends with the signing of the surgical consent form with the resident. In the case of major surgery may also include an explanation from a senior surgeon.

At the pre-op clinic Aaron was quiet and introverted, so Leah volunteered to tell me the sequence of events, which began three months earlier. She told me that Aaron

13

was a hard-working and dedicated taxi driver. They had three daughters—Aaron's pride and joy—two of whom were pregnant, and how he was looking forward to being a grandfather. He had always suffered from heartburn and thought it was work related— evening drives, unscheduled rides and sometimes night shifts. She had warned him that smoking like a chimney didn't help his condition. In the last three months the situation had worsened with frequent heartburn, upper abdominal pain and mild weight loss. At first, the family doctor didn't attach much importance to this and only changed Aaron's medication and scheduled a visit for a month later. At that follow-up, when the doctor saw that Aaron had lost even more weight, he recommended an emergency gastroscopy, and a huge tumor was found in Aaron's stomach. She remembers this day in great detail, because from that moment their lives were divided into 'before' and 'after'. She recalled Aaron waking up in recovery and the doctor informing them of the tumor and the biopsies, the shock that gripped them, the slow walk to the car and the roller coaster that followed: a chest and abdominal CT, an appointment with an oncologist, the biopsy results that confirmed malignancy, and the decision to have preoperative chemotherapy to reduce the size of the tumor.

During those three months Leah carried an organized binder and sat next to Aaron in meetings with the doctors. She met more doctors during that time than she had met her entire life. She and Aaron had their own in-jokes about the medical staff: the arrogant oncologist who talked to them in incomprehensible speech with lots of vague terms, and the secretary, who gave Aaron a pitying look when he told her he needed stickers for his day hospitalization in the oncology unit, and then blurted out, "Heaven forbid," when he told her about the tumor.

All this time together brought Aaron and Leah closer and increased their interdependence. Leah, who over the years had leaned on Aaron for everything, was now in charge, taking care of the house, the girls and her husband.

Dr Vasser also spoke to Aaron and Leah at the pre-op clinic and explained the complexity of the surgery and the complications that may follow. Since the tumor was close to the esophagus, he would have to perform a complete gastric bypass, remove all the surrounding lymph nodes and send them to pathology. He drew a sketch of the abdomen, esophagus, duodenum and small intestine and further explained that he would connect the esophagus to the small intestine, and after about a week, if there were no surprises, Aaron could go home and continue oncological follow-up. Later, Leah told me that she had heard what Dr Vasser said regarding possible severe post-operative complications, but his words hadn't registered with her, hadn't sunk in.

Our chief resident, Dr Shpet, who happens to be with me today as my senior resident, is also updated on Aaron's condition.

"There is pancreatic fluid in his drain," Puta tells Shpet, who enters Aaron's room with a toothpick between his teeth. Shpet has almost completed his residency and is about to become a senior surgeon. We all walk around in awe of him, a little afraid that he will humiliate us over a bad decision or a wrong move we make in surgery. Shpet attended Aaron's surgery a week ago, and he knows Aaron and his wife well. He leaves the room to talk to Dr Vasser, and tells me to return to the round.

Surgical residents don't actively participate in total gastrectomy until the end of their residency. The first couple of years are pretty bleak, fraught with difficult and frustrating moments on the ward, endlessly writing discharge letters and generally trying to keep our heads above water. They listen intently as senior residents recount heroic stories as the operating surgeon, such as: *I removed the tumor on my own; I performed the surgery skin-to-skin; It was a difficult gallbladder, but I removed all of it by myself.* On hearing these accounts, new residents shrink in the corner of the residents' room and wait for the day when they too will tell heroic stories. But as the years progress, residents do more and more. They start with small surgeries—the removal of a small lump in the skin; a subcutaneous biopsy; the removal of a port. I myself practice at home by suturing grapes and banana peel with surgical thread, tying knots on the girls' dolls and stitching badges on scout uniforms. Imrish sits with me in the seminar room and shows me exactly how Dr Kleiman likes the skin sutured.

"Here," he says, "take the thread, and instead of making an Aberdeen knot at the end, leave it and put steristrips over it."

He patiently watches me suture a piece of frozen chicken.

"Great," he says encouragingly, "now do it like that with Kleiman and he'll be over the moon."

I watch Aaron and Leah until they are no longer in sight as I continue the round. Dr Shpet is explaining Aaron's surgery to the interns, the words flowing from his mouth like melted butter.

"We removed the stomach, then performed an anastomosis of the jejunum to the esophagus, and lymph node dissection. One of the things that can occur when we do such a dissection around the pancreas, is a pancreatic leakage, and that's what we're seeing in Aaron's case." Shpet's eyes sparkle as the interns lap up his every word. "And what am I afraid of?" he asks rhetorically, before answering his own question. "I'm afraid he'll start bleeding, because pancreatic juice corrodes everything around it, including large blood vessels in the area." The interns nod silently, and as I laboriously continue typing, I am thankful that Aaron and his wife didn't overhear this conversation.

I slowly progress from one patient to the next, craving coffee. On a long shift, like today, I can drink 10 cups, not including the coffee on the ramp. The ramp is the parking area behind the hospital from where hospital orderlies transport patients for tests around the hospital. My residency colleagues and I go to the ramp to unwind over coffee and a cigarette, but mostly to re-energize each other—like the pink 'energon cubes' in the TV series *Transformers*—and breathe new life into another exhausting day on the 'battlefield'.

Our ramp ritual not only enables us to keep up-to-date with the condition of our patients and divide urgent tasks among us, it also gives us an opportunity to vent our anger, frustration and sadness, or just chat. It is one of the most enjoyable rituals of my surgical life, but the best ritual of all is undoubtedly the celebratory breakfast that residents prepare for the entire department after they perform a surgery for the first time, whether an appendectomy, a splenectomy or a cholecystectomy. The celebration is usually dedicated to the attending surgeon who supervised the surgery.

My congratulatory breakfast took place after my first laparoscopic appendectomy on a young, melancholy woman in her early twenties, who had to wait for surgery until early evening because the OR was busy in the morning. All the senior residents had already gone home, and I stayed behind, like a tiger lying in wait for its prey, knowing that this was my chance to perform my first surgery.

"A good surgeon is a hungry surgeon," Shpet once said to me, while he chewed on a fancy sandwich. "You have to constantly want to operate, to run after surgeries, to stay behind after everyone else leaves." So, I stayed behind and prepared for my first laparoscopic appendectomy together with the attending surgeon. The patient was anesthetized and I held her hand just before she fell into a dreamless sleep. I wondered if she could sense my apprehension and inexperience. But as I scrubbed in and looked in the mirror, something in me changed and I suddenly saw myself as a different person. Who is this surgeon with the glasses and surgical mask and hat? Perhaps she can be trusted after all.

I made the first incision, inserted the camera and the laparoscopic instruments, then grasped the inflamed appendix and slowly removed it, at the pace of someone doing it for the first time.

7 a.m.

During the round, as my hands alternate between examining patients and typing, my phone beeps. It's Tamar.

Mom, I don't have a white shirt for the ceremony at school today. Ahmed, the intern who is accompanying us on the round, asks me a question but I am distracted. I text Tamar: *Take a shirt from my closet.*

Fine, she replies, *but I told you yesterday mom!* Luckily, she ends the correspondence with a smiley emoji and a red beating heart. I set aside my feelings of guilt and disappointment in myself and refocus my attention on the round.

My daughters have numerous WhatsApp groups that I am randomly exposed to. For instance, Nitzan's second grade group was updated about a school event this coming Friday, and every family had to bring refreshments and text what they were bringing. With not enough time to juggle everything, I regretfully left it to the last minute and ended up having to bring sliced fruit. And now the white shirt for Tamar's ceremony. Yesterday she had said something to me on her way to the kitchen, and I nodded, but my mind was distracted, as always.

The girls remember the days when I was more at home. It was a bright period in my life. In the mornings I would swot up for the final exams before internship, then pick up the girls in the afternoon, Tamari from school, Nitzan from daycare, and come home to the warm smell of cooked pasta. I miss the calmness and quietude of those days, and when I look at old photos of the girls sitting playing after lunch or sitting in front of the TV eating grapes with their small hands—clearly happy that Mom is home—my heart truly aches. Nowadays, I occasionally get home from work by early afternoon, but I am so tired that I fall asleep with the newspaper in my hand. And the little energy I do have is often wasted on the residents' WhatsApp group following a report about some problem on the ward. So, although I am physically at home, my mind is often elsewhere.

When the girls and I do spend time together, they love to listen to stories about my patients. Nitzan collects letters I bring home and pastes them into an album, and Tamar gets excited when I receive gifts from my patients. And sometimes I think to myself that maybe this is enough, but I'm never quite sure.

"Dreznik," Puta growls at me, "we're heading to room 9, move yourself." I place the phone back in my pocket and drag Ahmed and the laptop with me. Room 9, or Cape Canaveral as we coin it, is like a mini-ICU on our ward that is usually occupied by the sickest patient, who will sooner or later 'launch' into a better place in the next world, or into the ICU when there is a slim chance to save them.

Room 9 is relatively spacious. It contains a ventilator and a monitor, and lying there now is Shoshana, intubated and in critical condition. She recently celebrated her 80th birthday and a few days ago came to the ER with severe abdominal pain. She had all the possible risk factors—diabetes, hypertension and arrhythmia—for mesenteric ischemia. In general surgery there are several events which are life-threatening if not immediately treated, including abdominal bleeding, free air in the abdominal cavity and mesenteric ischemia, which is like the cardiac infarction of the abdomen. Very often in cases of mesenteric ischemia we open the abdomen and find that most of the small intestine is already, or almost, necrotic because of a clot that has blocked the mesenteric artery responsible for its blood supply.

In Shoshana's case the situation was similar, however, enough of her small intestine could be saved, so we didn't remove all of it and in the reoperation our optimism paid off. Nevertheless, Shoshana was a very ill 80-year-old, who was unable to wean herself off artificial respiration, and we needed to move her to intensive care. Puta begins to dictate her condition to us: "A week after small bowel resection and reoperation with an ileostomy, ventilated, no evidence of spontaneous breathing." And out of the corner of my eye I see Imrish calling Golan, our on-call ICU physician. Imrish leaves the room for a moment and begs Golan for a bed in intensive care.

"Golan, Shoshana is maintaining blood pressure, we removed about a 100 cm of small bowel, she has a chance. Come and assess her." Imrish ends the conversation and returns to the room, his eyes conveying real concern, something we all feel for our patients. But Imrish is particularly concerned because Shoshana is his patient, whom he saw in the ER and operated on at 3 a.m. with a senior physician. He's the guardian angel of Shoshana's family; two sons, a daughter and a Filipino nanny who stay by her side around the clock and hang on Imrish's every word.

"Once you operate on a patient, they are yours for life," Shpet once told me in one of our first conversations at the start of my residency after he had helped me with the appendectomy of a patient who happened to be a nurse at our hospital. "It's surgical ethics," he added, looking deep into my eyes in earnest. "It means, Dreznik, that if a patient you operated on develops post-operative complications, you have to show up here to find out what happened, and if he's not well, you don't leave him. You lay down your life for him. That's what I expect of you.

A few days later I found out that the nurse we'd operated on was still hospitalized and in pain. It was a rainy Saturday morning and I raced to the hospital because I was worried there had been some complication in the surgery. The girls came with me and the three of us ran under an umbrella, dodging the puddles in the parking lot. When we arrived, my patient was sitting in a chair and I was relieved to hear that she was feeling much better. Yet it wasn't until she was discharged that I was able to relax and breathe normally again.

This was the first time I felt I couldn't breathe out of genuine concern for a patient. In the physician's oath there is a pledge that only then did I fully understand: "You will fully serve human life from its emergence from the mother's womb and the welfare of humans will unceasingly be your ultimate consideration." *Your ultimate consideration.* In medical school no one talks about the concern and fear that accompanies a doctor's life, yet it is there from the first intravenous infusion we administer and with every procedure we do on our own for the first time, the level of fear escalates. Sometimes when the fear overwhelms me, I remember what my uncle,

Prof. Dreznik, used to say: "A good surgeon should always be a little fearful, and his work should be treated with reverence. But only a little, because fear is paralyzing."

I glance at the clock, it's already 7:30 a.m. and there are still many more patients to get through. Puta needs to hurry to his first surgery of the day, Imrish is scheduled for consultations at the ambulatory clinic and I need to finish examining patients, write discharge letters and schedule special examinations, not to mention the lumpectomy I have with Dr Kleiman. But first I must get the trauma pager because I'm on-call today. Shept, as if reading my mind, suddenly arrives with it, and I shove it in my pocket and continue the endless round with the interns. I see on the laptop that I have six discharges, one of them to the ICU; there is an available bed for Shoshana. I breathe a sigh of relief.

No sooner have I finished the round than my pager beeps, as though the man upstairs had seen me put it in my pocket and decided to challenge me, just when I think I have a few moments to breathe. I tell the interns that I would not have survived all the day's tasks without them, and return the laptop to the charging station. Today, Ahmed is on ward duty and he must stay focused, especially now that Shoshana has been transferred to intensive care. Aaron, with the cloudy drains, is now the patient in the most serious medical condition, and Ahmed knows that he needs to take blood samples at noon, monitor his condition from time to time and notify me and Shept if his condition worsens. The pager beeps again and the voice of Bat-El, the nurse from the ER, emanates from it: "A serious road accident involving a pedestrian, a young woman of about twenty on the way here. Head, chest, abdominal injuries; in critical condition." As I listen to Bat-El, I see Shpet standing in front of me and hearing the exact same thing. We both run to the trauma unit. As a rush of adrenaline fills me, I hope this ends well, but I am skeptical. Based on the nurse's description, it seems like a very serious hit.
"It sounds like a thoracotomy, don't you think?" I ask Shpet.
"It sounds bad, Dreznik," he replies, "very bad."

8 a.m.

It takes forever to get to the trauma unit. First the stairs, then a long corridor at the end of which is the ER, by which time I am almost out of breath. Dr Klein, our trauma surgeon, once remarked: *I don't run to the trauma unit because I have to, but because I don't want someone else to get there before me*. Shpet and I keep running until we're finally there.

On the bed is a young woman, unconscious and breathing, and I immediately observe a huge hematoma on her left abdomen and car-tire marks on her legs. In TV shows, trauma unit activity looks so efficient, the medical staff ready-and-waiting with a syringe and defibrillator in hand. But in reality, there is total chaos. There are eight other medical staff in the room with me: four nurses, Shpet and Johnny—another surgical resident from my ward—three emergency medicine doctors, an anesthesiologist and Amir, the attending trauma surgeon, who orders an emergency thoracotomy. It's clear to us there is a very slim chance of saving her. Shpet announces that he is about to open the chest and the nurses open the thoracotomy set. Everything happens so fast. Within seconds, Shpet makes an incision from the middle of the chest to the left, exposing the heart, which isn't beating. A massive transfusion protocol is started, with large amounts of blood transfused through a central line at a dizzying pace as Shpet pumps the heart with his hands to fill it with blood. He then places the defibrillator on the exposed heart and manages to regain a pulse for a few seconds, before everything collapses again. After a few more resuscitation attempts, we eventually stop. The moment a person leaves the world of the living, there is always a few seconds of silence in the room. Amir looks at me and Johnny.

"Come," he says, "I want to teach you how to do cross clamping of the aorta." Aortic cross clamping is a procedure that can increase cardiac output and maintain essential circulation to the heart. It is a difficult technique to perform that requires

23

inserting your hands deep underneath the heart muscle, posterior to the left lung, feeling the esophagus and reaching deep below to the aorta, on which a device is placed that stops the blood flow in it. In critical and rare moments, it can save the patient, so it's important to be familiar with the anatomy and the technique. I insert my hands deep, trying to feel the esophagus, and finally, deep inside, I reach what feels like the aorta. I glance at the swollen, lifeless face of the young woman, who an hour earlier was alive and well, and my immense gratitude goes out to her for my opportunity to learn, through the tragic loss of her life, how to open a chest, hoping that this gratitude alleviates what feels like a blasphemous act, as my blood-stained gloves that envelop her lifeless heart. I shed no tears now; that will come later.

In the past, after such an event, I would flee to another room, stairwell or dark place, breathe heavily, take off my glasses and stare at a point in space, pondering the transience of life. But even in that momentary escape, the urgency of surgical life did not leave me.

All around me there is background noise and a shocking scene of blood, ripped clothes, hollow infusion tubes and medical staff coming to cover the body. In all the commotion a dense, disorienting fog suddenly descend on me, preventing me from absorbing what just happened. And only after the fog disperses, maybe days later, am I able to read about the tragedy in the headlines: *Young Woman Dies after Head-On Collision with Semi-Truck.*

A similar incident happened with a soldier who came to us two months ago after a fatal motorcycle accident, and we knew that he had died the second we put drains in his chest and large amounts of blood gushed out. On the way home I saw a picture of his smiling face on the newscast, and I couldn't comprehend how it had all ended so suddenly. And at that moment, the tears flowed, gathering the fragments of my mind and putting them back together again to cope another day.

The nurses collect the deceased woman's personal belongings and place them in a plastic bag. It's a horrible ritual that I cannot be part of, and I look away as Jenny, the nurse, removes a pink and purple bracelet from the woman's arm and pulls a ring off her finger. I leave the room and carry on; my long shift is still ahead of me.

It's 8:45 a.m. and I hurry to the OR, trying to forget the horrors of the trauma unit and trying to suppress my thoughts of the young girl's family on their way to the hospital, their hearts full of hope. They don't yet know what I know, still unaware of the devastation that has just occurred. I'm not sure I would have the strength to talk to them right now. I would hope they hadn't yet arrived at the hospital so that I could escape the heart-wrenching encounter from which there is no turning back. But usually, by the time the surgeon leaves the trauma unit, the family is waiting, sometimes just the parents or the children, and other times a whole clan, whose broken cries fill the entire corridor.

It takes me back in time. About a month ago, in the middle of a commotion in the ambulatory clinic and with patients in critical condition on the ward, the trauma pager beeped, alerting me to a 15-year-old boy who had tried to commit suicide and was on his way to the hospital, intubated with anoxic brain injury. I ran to the trauma unit, and within a few minutes an ambulance arrived with the boy who, according to the paramedics, suffered from a minor depressive disorder and took pills. That day his mother and younger brother had returned home to find that he had tried to hang himself. When they lifted him down from the rope, he had no pulse, but when they started resuscitation, they managed to get his pulse back. When he was rushed to the trauma unit, I went to check on him. I saw a young, tall boy, connected to a ventilator, his pupils not responding to light and his breathing shallow, indicating brain stem injury. We made sure there were no further injuries and did a head and neck CT. Then I was informed that his parents were waiting outside. Our trauma nurse looked at me in despair.

"Yael, you'll have to talk to them because they're waiting, they want to know what's happening." It was pretty obvious to me and the nurse what was happening. This boy would probably continue his life in a head injury rehabilitation center, never communicating with his family again, and may even remain in a vegetative state his whole life. But there is a big difference between what I supposedly know and what I am about to say to the boy's parents. After all, I can't just drop this huge bomb without preparing them for it. I go out to meet the parents and see a worried mother and a gaunt father who are afraid to look me in the eye. They are clearly in shock. The mother explains to me with surprising composure that she found her son hanging from a rope just a few hours ago. I am pretty sure that she is in denial and hasn't fully absorbed the events of the last few hours. I explain to them that their son is now stable, that we do not yet know the severity of his head injury and only in the hours and days to come will we know more. In the meantime, he will be hospitalized in the pediatric ICU for further treatment. I wait for an opportunity to leave them.

In the OR I don my scrubs and meet Shani, my patient, who is scheduled for a lumpectomy. She is waiting anxiously with her husband in the pre-op room. I introduce myself and she smiles at me, revealing the deepest dimples I have ever seen. She is a 50-year-old architect and generally healthy. She has two daughters, one of whom is on her honeymoon in Barcelona and the other is waiting outside the OR. About a month ago, while taking a shower, she felt a lump in her breast and immediately knew she had to see a doctor. Within a day she had made an appointment with a surgeon and had a mammogram and ultrasound. The tests revealed a relatively small 2 cm tumor in her left breast. A subsequent biopsy revealed carcinoma, a malignant tumor.

I had quickly taken in all this information this morning at home, and it was only when I arrived on the ward that I saw in the surgery file at the nurses' station that I had been scheduled for Shani's surgery. Every morning the list of surgeries to be performed that day is published in the file and next to each surgery is the name of the resident who will attend that surgery.

This morning Puta is ecstatic: He is scheduled for a laparoscopic right hemicolectomy, and he hopes he will be allowed to do the whole surgery by himself. We already anticipate Puta's celebratory breakfast and Imrish teases him about it, requesting the same delicious food that Puta's wife prepared after his previous surgery. "Shut up," Puta snorts at him.

In my first year of residency I rarely appeared in the surgery file, but with time I appeared with greater frequency and I kept a record of the details of my surgeries on my personal laptop. At the end of my residency, in order to become a specialist in general surgery, I have to present my surgical syllabus—a list of all the patients I have operated on. Unlike internal medicine, surgery is a manual, hands-on profession, and ultimately the experience pays off. People think that all surgeons are born with good hands, but in truth most of us lie somewhere in the center of the Gauss Curve, and what determines how well we will perform surgery in the future is generally a function of the amount of experience we acquire, as is the case in most professions.

I glance at the clock again and text Dr Kleiman that we are going into the OR with Shani, which is code for: "Get ready to come." Shani looks at me apprehensively.

"Will Dr Kleiman be in the surgery?" she asks, and I reassure her: "He's on his way here, don't worry." I hold her hand, she kisses her husband goodbye, and we go into the OR with the anesthesiologist and the nurse. I can't help but hope that one day someone will ask: "Will Dr Dreznik be in the surgery?" But I know that that day is still a long way off.

9 a.m.

"So, Dr Dreznik, what do you know about the patient?" Dr Kleiman asks me, his eyes penetrating through the lenses of his glasses. What can I tell him? That my acquaintance with her amounts to five minutes on account of having read her medical file early this morning? That all I know is that she is an architect and has two daughters? That as I held her hand her husband looked at her with love and concern? I throw dry medical information out the window and arrange Shani on the operating table with her left arm raised at a 90-degree angle. I inject methylene blue into the nipple to identify the sentinel axillary lymph node. The anesthesiologist looks at the monitor and the nurse scrubs in for surgery.

"She has an intra-ductal carcinoma, a palpable mass on the left, about 2 cm in size. No family history of breast cancer," I inform Dr Kleiman. He nods and glances at the medical file.

"Did you know that she also has diabetes and takes insulin?" he asks me as he continues to examine the file, and for a second it seems as though he's just waiting to trip me up. In the past we have occasionally fallen into the trap of going to surgery without sufficient knowledge of the patient, usually due to time constraints. But no one cares that I have just come from an unscheduled tragedy in the trauma unit, or that I'm exhausted after the morning's endless round, or that I don't know if my daughter went to school today in a white shirt. In time, I learned that a surgeon cannot operate on a patient without knowing all his medical details.

"Yes," I reply, "the endocrinologist gave instructions regarding the insulin; I wrote them in the file." I have the impression—perhaps due to my overdeveloped imagination—that Dr Kleiman is smiling behind his mask. We both go to scrub in. I want to tell him that I am not well acquainted with Shani; not like a doctor should be acquainted with a patient before surgery. Yet I do believe that true acquaintance comes from within, and begins the moment I accompany my patient in the most difficult moments, when their heart descends into a bottomless pit upon hearing the words 'tumor', 'biopsy', 'malignant'. Only when my eyes meet a soul reflecting from the depths of pain and sorrow, can I really know my patient. Dr Kleiman seems to be reading my mind, and as I scrub my right hand and then my left hand, he looks at me with Septol squirting into his palms.

"You know, Shani came to me for a checkup three weeks ago...she felt a lump in her breast while showering. We did a quick biopsy at the institute and she was debating whether or not to tell her daughter, who was about to go on her honeymoon." Kleiman pauses, then continues. "I told her I'm in favor of telling the family, but it's her decision. I think of the family waiting outside and of Dr Kleiman's sensitivity, and I suddenly see him in a more positive light.

When I was a new resident, I joined the "big rounds" on the ward that our boss, the head of the department, attended every Friday with all the senior doctors, residents and interns. Clad in white robes, we silently following the boss into each room, lapping up every word he said. During one of these rounds, Puta reproached me.

"There's no such thing as not remembering your patient's details, Dreznik," Puta rebuked. And if the boss asks you the patient's preoperative albumin level, you'd better not stutter like you just did. Now get with it!"

Back then I didn't understand the subtleties when it came to what I needed to know and didn't need to know; what to focus on; how to present a patient; how to separate out what really matters from the plethora of information that surrounds a patient. After Puta's rebuke, more embarrassing rebukes followed, one of which occurred while I was in a major oncological abdominal surgery with Dr Vasser, whom I greatly respect.

"Do you know the branches of the gastroduodenal artery?" Dr Vasser asked me. My heart dropped to my stomach and awful memories of my anatomy exam came flooding back. I was well familiar with the anatomy of the abdomen and the duodenum, but at that particular moment I couldn't remember the details. "You can't come to surgery with me if you don't know these things, Yael," Dr Vasser sternly warned me, and I felt myself diminish, wanting to disappear altogether.

Gradually, I learned that every senior doctor has their own particular area of focus. The boss, for instance, liked to know the patient's general condition—are they able to climb the stairs? Is there a supportive family that can help after surgery? We, the younger residents, navigated these inescapable questions in the best way we could. We read cluttered medical files, memorized hemoglobin, electrolyte and albumin levels, scrutinized patients' surgical and anatomical details and tried not to drown in the process.

"Just keep your head above water," Shpet said to me one day, "and eventually you'll learn to swim."

This historical term 'operating theater' comes from the medieval period when surgeries were performed in a small amphitheater where a crowd of students watched the surgeries take place. The surgeons did not wear gloves, only a stained and dirty apron that protected them from the patient's blood and secretions.

It took me a while to understand the meaning of the OR in all its layers, but to someone looking on from the side it looks like a spectacular show. Medical students enter the OR for the first time only in their fourth year of studies, and it's a completely different experience from anatomy courses in the first year. Some students realize early on that it's not for them—the prolonged standing, frustrating and tiring surgeries that can go on for hours, noisy nurses, an irritated anesthesiologist, an angry surgeon, the smell of diathermy that burns living tissues, and the uncontrollable bleeding. I once participated in a limb amputation of a diabetic patient in critical condition. This was my first clinical rotation as a student in surgery, after four long months in internal medicine. I waited impatiently to get to the OR, to that special moment when the patient is put to sleep and his flesh is cut.

Unlike the other rotations during medical studies, general surgery rotation includes an introduction to the OR and assistance with surgeries. The students' preparation for the OR involves several steps, the first of which is to learn how to scrub in for surgery—the exact number of minutes to scrub your hands—how to wear the sterile gown and how to conduct yourself in the OR. The most exciting moment is when the student actually participates in a surgery and is exposed to an exclusive fellowship where he gains a small part in the world of surgeons.

On my first day in general surgery rotation, I stayed behind in the afternoon and joined orthopedic surgeons for an emergency surgery. We all wore special nose and eye protectors, and I was allowed to hold the oscillating saw to cut the bone. But at that moment I felt a heavy fog descend on the room and had difficulty breathing. I felt weak, unable to stand on my feet any longer. Luckily, I realized that I was very close to passing out. This incident made me wonder if I was cut out for surgery, but thankfully it was an isolated incident and never reoccurred.

I hold the scalpel over Shani's tumor in the left breast.

"We are operating on Shani Cohen, left breast lumpectomy, antibiotic prophylaxis was given, no known sensitivities," Dr Kleiman declares to the medical staff in a procedure called a preincision time-out. "Make an incision here," he points, and I slide the scalpel over the skin, then open the tissues with the diathermy. "Give me a Babcock," Dr Kleiman continues, and the nurse hands him Babcock forceps with which he catches what looks like the tumor tissue inside the breast. "Now take clear margins around the tumor, so that there are no positive margins," Kleiman instructs, and I work carefully with the diathermy, wrapping the tumor in layers of fat around it, trying not to damage the surrounding skin or take out too much tissue, yet enough to get the whole tumor out. Then I mark the tumor with silk thread—top and left—to enable the pathologist orientation of the lump, and we hand it over to the nurse who puts it in a formalin bottle. I help Dr Kleiman remove the sentinel lymph node from the axilla and together we close the skin. Dr Kleiman sews skillfully, the result of years of experience, while I sew at a slower pace but try to get a perfect result. We finish the surgery and take off our gowns while the anesthesiologist starts waking Shani.

31

"You operated very well Dreznik, now write an operative report," says Dr Kleiman briefly, "and call in the resident who's after you for the next surgery. I'll wait for you so that we can talk to the family together."

Shani's husband and daughter see us approach them and quickly get up from their chairs, looking tense and anxious.

"The operation went well," Dr Kleiman reassures them. "We removed the entire lump and also removed a lymph node from the armpit that looks fine. Shani has already woken up and is breathing on her own. Tomorrow, if there are no problems, she can go home." I smile at them, knowing that out of all this information they have really only heard the words: *removed entire lump, breathing on her own*. The husband shakes Kleiman's hand, then mine, allowing himself to smile, his eyes a little teary, and he hugs his daughter who also thanks us both.

"Coming for a smoke?" Johnny asks me, as I leave the OR after having written the report and changed back into my usual uniform. It's almost 10 a.m., but it feels like at least a day has passed since I woke up this morning. Johnny and I go to the ramp; I have a few more minutes to myself before returning to the chaos on the ward, followed by the chaos of the ER that begins at 4 p.m. Johnny is currently in intensive care rotation, a welcome respite from the hard work on the ward. He starts his day at 8 a.m. ...pure luxury. And in spite of what its name suggests, the ICU is relatively calm compared to the heavy workload on a surgical ward, so much so that among ourselves we call it the 'inactive' care unit.

"So did Shoshana come to you?" I ask Johnny, as we hastily gulp down our coffee and wave at the hospital orderlies sitting near us.

"Yes," he replies, "she's a strong woman, I think she'll pull through. It was hard this morning," he continues, referring to the tragic death of the anonymous woman, which again cuts through me like a knife. I silently nod, lost for words. Maybe later. Maybe never. My phone rings, it's Imrish.

"Dreznik, come to the clinics, it's manic here. Then we'll take on the ward." I get up, my three-minute break is over.

"We'll meet at the evening round and then in the ER," I say to Johnny, who will be on-call with me and Shpet.

"Be strong," he urges with his half-crooked smile that I like so much, "and remember...morning always comes."

10 a.m.

I sit down at the ambulatory clinic, turn on the laptop and wipe the dust off the keyboard. I have no time for thoughts because outside there are at least 10 people still patiently waiting to see me and Imrish is working hard in the room next to me. At home I keep a record on my computer of all my thoughts on everything I am going through during my medical life, and my residency in particular. This is how I unwind my soul and manage to lift it again to meet the next challenge. All of us are dealing with life's challenges—exhaustion, intrusive thoughts, difficult moments in the face of loss, tragic news—when everything is shrouded in a thick fog with no light of hope. This is why I write. I wonder what I will write after this shift and how many hastily written words will compete with my fatigue. But for now, I must focus on my patients. I call in patient number 47, who by now impatient has already peeked through the door.

Shelley enters the room, sits down and begins a two-minute monolog, during which I become acquainted with the most intimate details of her life—one of the most extraordinary aspects of being a doctor. Shelley is a little over 60 and slightly plump. She has recently been suffering from upper abdominal pain, but has no fever. Her stools are normal, she's not vomiting and is generally healthy. An ultrasound revealed gallstones which are probably the cause of her pain. She came to the clinic on the advice of her family doctor who recommended she see a surgeon. After a polite conversation in which she tells me how many children she has, that she is now a retired grandmother, and how I look too young to be a doctor, we move to the examination bed. Just as cardiologists use a stethoscope to 'feel' the lub-dub sound of the heart, surgeons use their hands to feel the gastrointestinal organs and identify cholecystitis—inflammation of the gallbladder—acute appendicitis or bowel obstruction. Shelley and I discuss the need for a cholecystectomy and I explain to her what she should expect and how we will proceed.

"You know," she tells me, bleary-eyed, "All my life I worked hard. I had a business, I was self-employed, and I didn't spend enough time with my husband. And just after I retired a year ago, he passed away and I didn't get to be with him the way I wanted. And now this surgery. Sorry for bringing this up here, but I've just remembered how much I miss him." I feel a suffocating tightness in my chest. As she wipes her tears with a handkerchief, I get up from my desk, walk over to her and hold her hand, trying to catch her eye. Five minutes earlier we were complete strangers, and now she is baring her soul to me, just as I bare *my* soul on the keyboard at home. In a few moments she will leave the room, and when we meet again for the surgery we will both remember this conversation and the moment we shared together.

I finish typing, print out a summary of the meeting and hand it to Shelley before she leaves. I reflect on Shelley's words and wonder if I will be with *my* family in the way I want. After thousands of shifts and on-call hours on weekends and holidays, will I regret not spending more time with my loved ones?

For quite some time I have wanted to accompany Tamar's class on a school trip. But the school doesn't usually notify us of a trip in time for me to request a day off from my crazy shift schedule. Luckily, last year, I had a window of opportunity to take a day off and join Tamar's class on a trip. I filled out the 'Accompanying Parent Form' and imagined Tamar giggling with friends on the bus and feeling proud of her mother for coming along, just as I felt when my parents had accompanied me on school trips. But then it rained and the trip was unfortunately canceled.

"So come next time Mom!" Tamar urged me, and I searched her face for disappointment, but all I saw in her eyes was my own disappointment reflected back at me. Could I have foreseen these moments when I applied to medical school? Life seemed to go so smoothly back then, free of potholes and Saturdays laden with blood, wounds and ORs. At such times I always ask myself the proverbial question: Why medicine?

"Why do you want to become a doctor?" the psychologist asked me during my personality assessment before I was admitted to Tel Aviv university's Faculty of Medicine ten years earlier. The meeting with the psychologist took place after simulations, role-plays and other interviews designed to identify best-fit medical students. I had rehearsed my answer to this question over and over at home in front of Gadi: *I want to be a doctor because I want to help people, treat them, save lives.* It sounded so pale and clichéd to me. The psychologist looked at me intently, perhaps looking for authenticity, and both she and I knew how fed up she was with the answers of hundreds of candidates who had repeated the same mantra. The words stuck in my throat as all my rehearsals vanished into thin air and a tense silence descended on the room. So, I told the psychologist a story about a little girl named Mor, whom I met while volunteering some years back for an organization that helped underprivileged kids. Mor was having difficulty at school and I was assigned to give her private lessons to help her with homework. Her family was struggling; her mother was very ill and her father was barely able to keep his head above water. On my first day with Mor, I drove—with much apprehension—to a poor and dilapidated neighborhood in the city. She was waiting for me at the entrance to her apartment building, a sweet girl, whose smile illuminated her gloomy home. She sat me down in the dining room and made me raspberry juice, then we started working on her homework. Her mother sat in a wheelchair, looking old and distant, and her father, whom I met for a split second, thanked me and left. He looked wrinkled and tired, just like the building they lived in. When I left, I cried uncontrollably. I told the psychologist of the purifying sensation that seeped into me following my act of giving, and a small tear rolled down my face. And that was my answer to psychologist's question.

My stomach rumbles and I remember that I haven't eaten since morning. Imrish and I are doing a good job of managing the clinic, and now seems like a good time to escape to the cafeteria, a two-minute walk away. But just then, at an inopportune moment, Smadar, patient number 51, enters the room. I immediately recognize her—a lovely woman whose appendix I had removed a month ago. Today she is here for follow-up. Smadar opens her arms to give me a warm hug, then hands me a big bar of chocolate. There are some patients who, even after we save their lives, are discharged home and barely say goodbye to the staff, and then there are others who feel eternally indebted to us for simply relieving their pain in the ER.

"Dr Yael, I'm so happy to see you!" says Smadar, smiling radiantly as she sits down. We chat for a while, then I examine her and am very pleased to see that the scars from the surgery have healed nicely. By this time, I am so hungry that I have no qualms about reaching for the chocolate she brought me, and I offer her some too. Suddenly my day seems brighter and I have a taste for more.

Between patients I run to the bathroom. My WhatsApp flashes and it's Miri, one of my best friends from medical school, who is now a pediatrician, working at a community clinic. *Yaeli, can I call? Need advice* her message reads. Friendships formed at medical school mature over the years into an offshoot consulting network. Occasionally I send Miri a picture of a skin rash and pick her brain about it, and sometimes she will confer with me about a surgical issue involving a neighbor or a friend. It's hard to explain how vital the pool of advice and guidance is at times. I take advantage of the few minutes of quiet I have to call her. Miri answers me immediately. She remembers how already in my fourth year of medical school I aspired to be a pediatric surgeon, and how ecstatic I was when I told her about the appendectomy of a small boy I attended. Since then, she shares all her surgical cases with me.

"I'm at the clinic," Miri says, "and there's a nine-month-old baby here named Yuval. The senior physician is with him. To cut a long story short, the baby has not stopped vomiting all morning and looks lethargic. The parents are really concerned. We suspect intussusception, so we referred him to the pediatric ER. Are you on duty today by any chance? " I answer in the affirmative.

"I'm stuck at the clinic right now," I reply, "but we'll probably be called to the pediatric ER after the baby has an ultrasound. Tell the parents to come to the ER straightaway." At the end of the conversation, I call the pediatric ER and inform one of the residents of the expected arrival of the baby.

I remember the first time I performed surgery for intussusception with Dr Shenhav, a pediatric surgeon. Intussusception is a serious condition in which one part of the intestine folds into another part like a telescope, causing intestinal obstruction, which if not opened in time, may lead to intestinal necrosis, putting the baby in a life-threatening condition. As I end my conversation with the ER, I imagine a gun appearing in Act 1 of this drama, knowing deep down that there will be a shot in Act 3... but I still have time.

11 a.m.

With our work at the ambulatory clinic behind us, Imrish and I return to the ward and I, in mild hyperglycemia, shove three rows of the chocolate bar into my mouth. Considering the long, stressful hours doctors work, with little time to eat, coupled with cumulative fatigue, one would assume that they would lose weight, but the exact opposite is true. God knows how many cheese toasts I've eaten in the middle of the night, how many vending machine potato chips I've consumed because I didn't have time to eat a nutritious meal, how many trays of pizza I and my colleagues have polished off in the small hours of the morning to keep us awake. This creates a situation where the ward's moving average in terms of weight gain is always positive. Dr Shpet's pot belly, for instance, is a classic resident's belly that developed after years of hard work and uncontrollable overeating in two main areas of the hospital: the kitchen in the pediatric building where the food is really good, and the radiologist's room where there is always tasty food in colorful plastic containers which we eat after getting partial permission.

"What else needs to be done on the ward?" Imrish asks me, as we climb the stairs because the elevators are busy. I'm a little out of breath due to the chocolate I've just eaten and also the fact that I'm really out of shape.

"There's still the discharge letters to write," I gasp. "It remains to be seen how Bergman will be presented for rehab, and Yanai for complex nursing. Today I only have approval for two abdominal CT scans so far. Dr Clinger hasn't approved a chest and abdomen CT for Alexei with the metastasis; she says it isn't urgent. Oh, and we need to check up on Roth in room 5, see how his colonoscopy went." Imrish nods, holding a bag of savory pastries he bought this morning on his way to the clinic, which are now cold and tasteless.

"Remind me again...what's the story with Bergman?" Imrish asks. "And how exactly are we going to present him for rehab?"

I first met Mr. Bergman in the ER a few days ago. I didn't know then that he would become a 'frequent flyer' and be repeatedly admitted to the hospital. He was a former engineer, had two children and led a fairly normal life. He used to have one stiff drink a day, but following his dismissal from his job he got addicted and consumed excessive amounts of alcohol that messed up his liver. As a result, he suffers from cirrhosis—an advanced stage of scarring of the liver tissue with a poor prognosis—which caused varicose veins to form in the esophagus. Varicose veins are the medical term for swollen, enlarged and dilated veins, which usually appear in the lower end of the esophagus or in the upper stomach. The clinical presentation of bleeding from these varicose veins is dramatic—a patient who vomits large amounts of fresh blood in the ER is quickly admitted to the shock room for an emergency gastroscopy.

This was the case with Bergman when he was brought to the ER, and I still have a small blood stain on my shoe from all the drama that went down in the shock room with him. Bergman had been found alone on the street in severe neglect with overgrown fingernails and wreaking of alcohol. We had almost no medical history of him. His ex-wife, who was still caring for him, told us about the months of uncontrollable drinking and self-destructive tendencies. A gastroscopy revealed some bleeding varicose veins that had been ligated by the gastroenterologist, so he was admitted to our ward with full monitoring, blood transfusions and treatment to lower his blood pressure and prevent the veins from suddenly bleeding again.

Back on the ward I go to check on Bergman and notice that his eyes are light blue, almost transparent. As I talk to him he looks at me, but he seems to be in another place that I have no access to. His children don't visit him and most of the time he's alone, caressing the white stubble on his face with his long nails, looking sad and defeated. His ex-wife comes occasionally with some food, even though he still needs to fast, and she exchanges a few words with the staff. The day Bergman was admitted to the ward she approached me.

"You have to help me wean him off alcohol," she pleaded, "he's killing himself." I saw that she cared. They probably had some good years of family life and a relationship that is now completely destroyed.

"We've never dealt with alcohol rehab on the ward, we're a surgical ward," I tell her. However, at noon I called a psychiatrist at the hospital to ask his opinion, and he gave me the phone number of a rehab center in the hospital with an organized clinic and follow-up. I had a feeling that Bergman wouldn't be going to this rehab center. During my conversation with him he had looked pale and hollow-eyed, his mind shattered from months of deterioration, and perhaps he was waiting to be discharged so he could go back to drinking. But in the meantime, he's still here with us.

Bergman has joined a long list of patients I would never have met in any other job, the kind my non-medical friends have. This list includes street prostitutes who come to the ER completely drugged, with bruises all over their bodies, cursing and causing a commotion, and drug smugglers, who have swallowed cocaine capsules or inserted them into their rectum, and are brought to the ER under tight security after being arrested at the airport. Mostly these are unemployed middle-aged people who were tempted to make easy money from drug dealers at the cost of risking their lives—because no one told them that the release of pure cocaine in the stomach can cause cardiac arrest and a quick death, as happened once when a drug smuggler died shortly after arriving at the ER in critical condition.

Sometimes I had to examine prisoners who arrived in handcuffs and leg restraints, in pain and in bad general condition, with guards watching over them, not allowing them any privacy during a physical examination. Once, while I was examining a prisoner, I was told that he used to rape his daughters. I couldn't look at him or touch him, and averted my eyes from him in disgust, thankful after the examination that I would never have to see him again. Since then, I have maintained a distance between me and these patients and try never to ask questions unrelated to the medical condition itself.

I have also seen neglected and abused children in the ER, as well as battered women from all racial and ethnic groups, with black eyes, ruptured spleens, or cuts all over their body, which I sutured with tears in my eyes, bitterly angry at the evil in the world and frustrated at how small I am in comparison to it, unable, in most cases, to change anything. Bergman joined this long list of sad patients, again underscoring the limitations in our ability to cure everyone, like a loose band-aid on a bleeding wound. And yet, in Bergman's discharge letter today I recommended follow-up at an alcohol detox clinic, as if the words, written in black and white, held a solemn promise for the future.

It's almost noon and the ward is full of visitors. The nurses are scurrying around the patients with medications and infusions, and our interns are working hard, like doped ants, on the mountain of tasks we left them to do. As for me, a whole life has gone by in the last few hours, during which I was involved in an unsuccessful attempt to save the life of a young traumatized woman; operated on Shani with the breast tumor; and received patients at the ambulatory clinic. Ahmed, the intern, is in room 11, trying to insert an IV into the arm of a patient who is getting impatient, asking him to call another doctor. I see the look of frustration in Ahmed's eyes, the frustration we all feel when we fail at the smallest thing like inserting an IV. It can cripple us, leaving us feeling incompetent and inadequate.

"I'll ask Dr Dreznik," Ahmed tells the patient, and she smiles sourly at me.

"I really hope you'll succeed," she says to me, "I've no veins left because of you lot." I sit down in front of her with a quiet sigh and look at all the needle marks from Ahmed's numerous attempts at finding a suitable vein in the arm of this particularly difficult patient. After a laborious search I find a tiny vein next to the socket of the arm. I am congratulated on my success and feel very proud of myself, but I know I could just as easily have failed.

"She has no veins, I could barely find one," I say to Ahmed, in an attempt to make him feel better and restore his confidence. I try to convey to him that our world is far from perfect and that sometimes we have to hold on to each other in order to feel our worth. We all fail as doctors; it's part and parcel of this profession, but you can get through it with the small successes along the way. Out of the corner of my eye I see Ahmed approach Aaron and take several blood samples. I peek at the drains, happy to see they are not bloody and pray that Aaron will be okay. My phone beeps, it's a message from Puta: *Dreznik, do me a favor, I have a student lesson in ten minutes, but I just now got out of surgery and have to finish a presentation for the boss. Fill in for me...do a teaching case with them.* I catch my breath, calculate my chances of grabbing something to eat, text Imrish, telling him to take care of the rest of the tasks until the evening round, then glance at Aaron, who looks at me with his lovely, quiet smile. I smile back at him.

Noon

It's 12:05 p.m. The sun is at its highest point in the sky, but here on the ward neon lighting dominates and only a warm summer breeze drifts through the window in one of the rooms as a brief reminder of the world outside. Puta is working on his presentation for the boss, Imrish is running around doing a million task, and I have to contend with an unplanned students' lesson and break my head over what to talk to them about that will impart something of value from my relatively little knowledge about general surgery.

Shortly before the start of my residency I took Nitzan and Tamar to the sea one summer morning on a spur-of-the-moment decision. The beach was unusually empty for the middle of July. The girls made sandcastles and jumped into the waves, occasionally glancing over at me to check that I was there, present in the moment of our time alone. I tried to give a name to that moment...an unimpeded moment before I would become a specialist in a very demanding profession. I tried to formulate for myself rules to live by, rules for work, for motherhood, and above all to breathe in the moment, the smell of the salty sea filled with a lot of questions.

One of most daunting transitions in a doctor's life is the transition from resident to specialist. This is when your formal medical training ends and The Ministry of Health sends you a medical specialist license. And that's it—you're on your own from now on. No more passing the buck; your patients' treatment is your responsibility, and yours alone.

The transition from internship to residency is no less daunting to me. Residents can write prescriptions, discharge patients, decide on hospitalization. Sometimes I don't even realize the responsibility I hold, and I'm not yet a specialist. I dwell on this as I make my way to the lesson, wondering how I can convey to the students this sense of responsibility for human life. They aren't there yet, but it won't be long before things around here are on their watch.

Six fourth year medical students are waiting for me in the conference room. They currently accompany doctors on surgical ward rounds. Puta is their tutor and he will be in charge of them during the two months they will be with us on the ward. Medical studies are divided into two main parts—the pre-clinical years at university when students learn physics, chemistry, anatomy, physiology and the human body systems, and the clinical years, when they are assigned to university-affiliated hospitals. They undergo training in all of the hospital's main departments: internal medicine, general surgery, pediatrics, anesthesia, psychiatry, gynecology and so forth. On the first day of their clinical years, students learn basic skills—how to take blood, how to do an ECG and interpret its reading, how to perform a physical examination, starting with a neurological examination, listening to the heart, examining the chest, breasts, abdomen and ending with a rectal examination.

I remember the first time I tried to take blood from the femoral vein of a patient on the internal ward. The patient was lying down, legs slightly apart. I touched the inside of her thigh and felt the femoral artery throbbing. I took a syringe with a green needle, then disinfected the groin with an alcohol pad, my heart racing. I had to try to navigate the vein without piercing the artery, and I needed to go deep. I gently inserted the needle, but then stopped, too afraid to go deeper. The senior doctor next to me took over and skillfully went deeper at a slightly different angle, and in a split second the test tube filled with blood. How I longed to be her at the moment; to wear a white coat like the other doctors on the ward and take blood as easy as pie. I yearned for nothing but to learn how to become a doctor.

The medical profession is an apprenticeship, an art, acquired after many years of training, experience, and a lot of blood, sweat and tears to make it through. Like any apprenticeship occupation, medicine is a hierarchical system and reveres the experience of senior doctors who guide and teach residents the ropes of the profession. General surgery is particularly difficult because it requires manual skills that take many years to develop, as well as the ability to make decisions in the OR: when to operate, when to wait, when not to take a risk. As a senior doctor in the department once told me: "During my years of residency I learned how to operate. Then when I became a senior doctor, I learned who should not be operated on." In the hospital's ecosystem, medical students are the most valued and most invested resource. The opposite holds true for interns, who are at the bottom of the medical hierarchy and do most of the menial work, serving as modern day slaves, despite the fact that they have already spent years in medical school. But this is how the wheels keep turning...

"Have you already done a teaching case?" I ask the students, as I sit down at the head of the conference table in the boss's seat, wondering to myself how many more years would pass before I'd have the opportunity to sit at the head of the table. The students stare at me, sitting with their cups of coffee and boxes of home-cooked food, just as I did a few years earlier. Before coming to the conference room, I was updated that Bergman had vomited blood, and it latches onto my brain, robbing me of a quiet mind. I look at the students, a little envious of their serenity and aloofness. After this lecture, they will have the luxury of going home to a tranquility I wish I could escape to.

One of the students, a sweet red-haired girl, informs me they do not know what a teaching case is. The rest smile shyly at me and wait, pens ready, for me to explain.

"In a teaching case I present you with a true medical scenario and ask you questions, and this is how you learn something new. For instance, have you been taught how to do an abdominal examination?" I ask, and they nod. "Fine, so let's tell a story. Michal," I say, turning to the redhead, "you are now a surgeon in the ER and an 80-year-old man arrives. He suffers from dementia and hypertension and he's taking aspirin and other medications to balance his blood pressure. He's been vomiting all morning. His caregiver, who has come with him to the ER, noticed some blood in his vomit. What's the first thing you do?"

Michal looks at me, focused. The rest of the students begin to wake up, they too are alert. Students don't really understand that the day will come when someone turns up at ER in a life-threatening condition, and in a split second they will have to put all their theoretical knowledge into practice.

"I first take vital signs and ask the nurse for blood samples," Michal replies, and I nod. She appears to have tenacity and good surgical intuition. She describes the lab tests she asks for, and then I stop her and move on to the student next to her, a tall, swarthy guy with glasses.

"Amos, right?" I ask. I remember that in the opening discussion a week earlier he had said he wanted to go into internal medicine, probably cardiology. "Amos, it's your turn. The lab tests Michal asks for are in the works, the patient is slightly tachycardic, his blood pressure is maintained and he has no fever. How do you continue from here?" Amos looks at me, thinking what to say.

"I think if he's vomiting blood then there is suspected gastric bleeding, so it seems to me that an emergency gastroscopy is in order," Amos replies.

"What about a physical examination?" I ask him, and he stutters a little, realizing that he hasn't handle the case properly, that first you have to examine the patient before deciding what to do.

"Obviously I do a physical examination, lift up his shirt, examine his abdomen," Amos replies. I ask him what exactly he wants to examine. Amos hesitates, then says, "I want to know if there is abdominal swelling or tenderness for example."

"The abdomen is not swollen, maybe very little, and there is no tenderness," I respond. Amos keeps answering, trying to aim for what I want him to say.

I remember the *real* man who came to the ER about a year ago and whom we almost lost. Exactly the same story, only in real life. It was a Friday morning and Puta and I were informed of a 90-year-old man who was vomiting coffee-ground vomitus. We went to his cubicle and tried to take an anamnesis and ask him how it all started, but since he had dementia and was uncooperative, it was very difficult. His foreign caregiver told us in broken English that he had vomited a few times and was taking several medications. In a case like this, which is similar to examining a baby who can't tell you what's bothering them, it's extremely important to do a physical examination to try to

47

figure out the cause of the symptoms and how to proceed with treatment. Puta and I almost forgot to do the most important thing in an abdominal examination: remove the grandfather's pants. When we did this, we discovered swelling in the groin—a strangulated, stiff, rather small and unmistakable femoral hernia, which caused an intestinal obstruction, then vomiting which led to hematemesis,[1] and there was no choice but to proceed to an urgent surgery.

Amos, the student, continues to ask for a gastroscopy, and I, having no choice, try my luck with Rachel, a diligent-looking student who's waiting for my next question.

"Rachel, Amos asks for a gastroscopy and you happen to be the on-call gastroenterologist. Amos fills you in on the patient's condition. What can you tell me about the differential diagnosis of hematemesis in an adult?" Rachel fires all the answers that come to her mind, from a gastric ulcer and a vascular malformation to tumors and intestinal obstruction. I glance at the clock. Half an hour has gone by since I presented the case, and through the open door of the conference room I see Puta, on his way back from the surgery, winking at me in the hallway. He had obviously done the entire surgery himself and I am wholeheartedly happy for him.

Eventually, Michal, the redhead, comes up with the correct answer: To remove the grandfather's pants and check his groin for a strangulated hernia, which doesn't require a gastroscopy, but an urgent surgery. Amos looks down, but he will remember this lecture, because it is from our mistakes that we learn the most, and I cannot help but think about my very first 26-hour on-call shift.

---

[1] Vomiting of blood.

1 p.m.

About three years ago, in the early hours of a sunny May morning, I left home for my first 26-hour on-call shift at the hospital as an intern on the internal ward. I carried a tattered backpack from our recent trip to New Zealand with the girls, which still had the nostalgic smell of our caravan and the Pacific Ocean. That day the backpack was full of energy bars, some fruit, a toothbrush and toothpaste. This was the first time I would be in the hospital for more than 24 hours, the first time I would be pushed over my stress threshold when all the doctors had gone home and I and another resident would be left on our own to manage more than thirty patients. Nothing can prepare you for this; it's like waking up the morning after your first day in the army and realizing that you are in a different reality. Somehow you get through it, but you never forget the hallucinatory experience. Patients and their families often ask me about my shifts, questions such as: *What, you do shifts around the clock? How many hours have you been here? Have you really been here since yesterday morning?* Their questions indicate how uninformed they are about what doctors actually do. And understandably so, because let's face it, who can grasp the reality of a doctor's workload in a world where all other jobs have long since abandoned this inconceivable work model?

Luckily, my shift on the internal ward flew by with a million tasks to do. I took blood samples, did ECGs, accompanied unstable patients to the cardiology and imaging units and admitted new patients whom I presented to senior doctors. At 18:00, I sipped a cold coffee that I had made an hour earlier and got acquainted with Alex, a chubby patient with smiling eyes. He was a tour guide in his 60s who had arrived that day with severe pneumonia. He could barely breathe, had a high fever and his heavy cough only made it worse. His wife was by his side. I examined him and filled out his medical intake form.

Evening descended on the ward, and I and the resident on duty with me admitted two new patients—a young man who had attempted suicide and an elderly man with kidney failure. Besides that, there were two or three patients in poor general condition who needed re-examinations. Then night came and the nurse asked me to administer 4 mg of morphine to Alex intravenously. She handed me a syringe containing 10 cc of morphine, all of which I injected into Alex's vein and returned the empty syringe to her. The nurse gave me a worried look as she told me I should have only given Alex half the amount. I must have turned pale and my pulse rate jumped to 200 beats a minute and an overwhelming fear gripped me. *Dear God, what have I done? God, please make it okay.*

Engraved in stone at the entrance to Tel Aviv University's Faculty of Medicine where I studied, is the well-known edict 'First, do no harm', the bedrock of medical ethics. That evening I was struck with paralyzing fear for Alex's life. The resident with me tried to calm me down and we immediately informed the toxicology lab of my mistake and told Alex that he had received a double dose of morphine, and that if he had difficulty breathing due to respiratory depression, we would give him an antidote that would counteract the effect of the morphine overdose.

I will remember that night forever. I was riddled with guilt and shame for making a disastrous mistake which could cost a human life. I only managed to fall asleep at 5 a.m. after checking on Alex every single hour to see that he was breathing and getting better. In the morning Alex requested that I give him the same dose of morphine again because he had finally managed to sleep and expel mucus and was feeling comfortable and happy. I began to relax and staggered home with aching legs, promising myself to be more careful in the future and double check everything.

After the lesson with the students, I tidy up the conference room, look for a file on the computer that I promised to send them, make a note of the tasks I still have to do on my shift, and wonder if the girls have already returned home from school. My phone rings.

"Dreznik, it's Shay, I'm in the pediatric ER. How are you?"

"I'm fine, what's up?" I reply, my phone on speaker as I scroll through my WhatsApp and see loads of messages on the residents' group that I haven't had a chance to respond to, while trying to figure out why Shay, a senior pediatrician, is looking for me. Then I remember baby Yuval, with suspected intussusception.

When Nitzan, my younger daughter, was about three years old, her daycare teacher called me in a panic and said that Nitzan looked lethargic and sleepy. I was in my sixth year of medical school at the time, and like any medical student the most awful scenarios ran through my head: meningitis, encephalitis, a brain tumor. That day I picked her up early from daycare. She had a fever, was very chatty, ate some chocolate and seemed alert.

But the report of Nitzan's teacher, whom I trusted implicitly, was disturbing. So Gadi and I took her to the ER where I met Shay, then a pediatric resident, who examined her and didn't seem particularly concerned. I was then on the other side of the fence, in the role of the worried and anxious mother in need of reassurance from someone I could trust. Once Nitzan's blood and urine tests were fairly normal, we were eventually discharged. I don't miss for one minute being on the other side of the fence, feeling utterly helpless, but I will never forget Shay and how he took good care of Nitzan in the ER. So, every time he calls and asks for surgical advice, I immediately answer and try to give him a timely and professional response.

"I have a baby here who is a few months old," Shay continues. "I did an ultrasound and it looks like intussusception. His name is Yuval Rabinovich. I'm sending him for an air enema, and I understand that you are on call. I'm also updating Dr Shenhav," Shay adds, and I jot down another task for later. "How's the shift so far?" he enquires. I smile into my phone, then leave the conference room and head towards the bustle on the ward.

"So far, so good," I reply with my usual answer and end the call. I make a note to myself to update Miri later on the fate of the baby, but that will only be when all this mess is over.

51

"Are we starting the evening round?" asks Puta irritably as he storms into the residents' room. It's 1:30 p.m. and now that I've I finished with the students and sent them to do admissions for some patients on the ward, I have a few minutes to spend with Imrish in the residents' room and quickly eat a sandwich and a packet of potato chips. The smell of Septol on my hands blends in with the oil in the potato chips, now deep in my stomach, but I know this food will hold me over the next few hours, like a soldier who opens a combat ration and eats it until he's full, because he doesn't know when he'll get a chance to eat again.

"What happened, was there a double scrub up?" I ask Puta with a chuckle, and he responds with a growl, cursing the interns who didn't have time to do all the tests he wanted done. Underneath Puta's growling and irascibility is a big heart, but he doesn't want everyone to know this fact. When his patients are in distress, he is devoted to them, and when he hears patients groan in the ER, he does everything in his power to relieve them of their pain. Above all, he protects us, his team, and won't let any one of us come to harm.

'Double scrub up' is an epithet we residents apply to a situation where two senior surgeons and a resident scrub in for a surgery, but the two surgeons perform most of the surgery while the resident looks on and only gets to minimally participate. At the start of residency this is understandable, since new residents still don't know how to operate, but Puta is already in the middle of his residency, has already sat his in-training exams, and was so looking forward to his first laparoscopic right colectomy, a significant part of our syllabus.

"Dreznik, don 't annoy me right now," Puta shoots. "We'll go to the ramp after we finish up this farce here," he adds and then continues: "Imrish, what the hell are we doing about Bergman's hematemesis? Have you updated the on-call gastro?" Imrish and Puta sit down at the computers next to me, and we carry out our quick and goal-oriented ritual of going over our entire list of patients, getting ready for this evening's big visit with our on-call surgeon and presenting the patients before nightfall.

"Ok, let's quickly go over the list," says Puta. "Ahmed, sit here next to us, you're looking after the ward today, so pay attention to all the asterisks."

'Asterisks' is our code name for the group of patients we need to keep a close eye on, the ones who can ruin our night if, for instance, they develop sepsis or respiratory failure.

"First of all, how is Aaron? What about his drains?" Puta asks. Imrish updates us that the drains are cloudy but Aaron is stable, has no fever. "Good," Puta says, eating Ferrero Rocher one after the other and washing them down with diet coke. "Ahmed, I want you to do lab tests again this evening, and update Dreznik on any problem, she's in charge of you." Ahmed nods, looking stressed. "Now, what about Mrs Roth's colonoscopy? Do we have the results?" I begin reading the colonoscopy report: *Multiple non-bleeding diverticula have been observed along the left colon, the rest of the colonoscopy is normal.* Puta looks at Mrs Roth's lab tests, which two days ago indicated bleeding, and instructs Ahmed: "Check with the hematologists when we need to renew her blood thinners. If it can wait, we will send her home tomorrow, and if not, we will renew them during hospitalization." Imrish updates us on the condition of Shoshana who moved to intensive care, and I continue to document consultations that we haven't had time to do since this morning. We finish going over the list when, in perfect timing, Dr Cohen, our on-call senior doctor, enters the room.

"This evening's round is with me and the red side at 3 p.m. prompt," he says, and leaves. Puta stares at me.

"Dreznik, do a quick walk through the trauma unit," he instructs me, "then we'll meet on the ramp for coffee. Come on, move it." I leave the hustle and bustle of the room, and as my on-call shift draws near, I start to feel on edge, as I did before my first on-call shift as an intern; the restlessness, the worry, the hope that the shift will end well.

2 p.m.

The trauma unit, which is a few meters from our ward, provides care for patients suffering from major traumatic injuries, such as stab wounds, motor vehicle collisions, falls, and so forth. The unit has several beds and the patients are closely monitored by a dedicated team of nurses and close supervision of our department.

In 1976, in the US state of Nebraska, orthopedic surgeon and amateur pilot, Dr James K. Styner, was flying home in his private aircraft when it crashed with his wife and four children onboard. His wife was killed instantly and three of the four children suffered severe head injuries. Styner and his son Chris suffered minor injuries and were able to evacuate the unconscious children from the aircraft. Not far from the scene of the accident, Styner managed to flag down a car with two travelers who took Steiner and his children to a hospital in the area. But when they arrived the hospital was closed, and once enough medical staff had been gathered to open it, Styner discovered that the doctors were unskilled in managing trauma. Luckily, he and all four children survived, but Styner realized that he himself had provided better care at the scene of the tragic accident than that provided to him and his children at the hospital, indicating that the system was seriously flawed and needed to change. Within a few years, Styner set up an entire system for trauma management in hospitals, and as part of its protocol it was decided that trauma cases, whether they involve a head injury, abdominal injury or an orthopedic problem, would be managed by general surgeons, an approach which has been adopted in many parts of the world.

This story led me to wonder how general surgery got its name. Perhaps it's because general surgery is so diverse and includes abdominal surgery, transplants, and the management of trauma patients.

Trauma management begins when the casualty arrives at the shock room and the trauma team must rapidly do a trauma assessment and prioritize treatment, for which there is a very orderly protocol. For instance, if a patient has a head injury and an abdominal injury, which is the most urgent to treat? Should we do a combined surgery? Should the intra-abdominal bleeding be treated before the head injury? And what about pregnant women or babies, whose physiological function is different from that of elderly people? What about a multi-casualty incident? Any number of scenarios can play out unexpectedly at any given moment.

I enter the trauma unit with the pager, which this morning updated me on the anonymous young women in the fatal road accident. Every time I am on-call, the pager hangs on my uniform like a kind of status symbol that sets me apart from the other residents at the hospital. In most cases, trauma injuries turn out to be relatively minor; a combination of several injuries to the limbs, head, chest and abdomen that require an imaging test, such as a whole-body CT scan, and there is usually no threat to the patient's life. The remaining injuries are either serious, requiring surgery and hospitalization in intensive care, or critical, for instance when the casualty sustains pelvic hemorrhage requiring pelvic packing in the shock room, or presents with tension pneumothorax or internal chest bleeding requiring immediate insertion of a chest drain or an emergency thoracotomy, as was the case this morning. In such cases there is always a lot of medical staff in the shock room, but only one person calls the shots—the attending trauma surgeon. He is the one who determines treatment and almost never treats the wounded himself but keeps an eye on the monitor to examines the condition of the casualty. My attending trauma surgeon, Amir, is waiting for me at the entrance to the trauma unit so that together we can discuss the patients who are hospitalized.

Our trauma unit usually consists of three to six patients with varying degrees of injury. Some of them will be discharged, while others have had emergency surgery, such as Anat in bed 6, mother to two little boys. About two weeks ago, while she was tidying a closet at home, one of the drawers fell on her and injured the upper left side of her abdomen. She was in pain but didn't attach much importance to it. Later that day, when she began to feel extremely weak, she knocked on her neighbors' door and fainted in front of him in the stairwell. The neighbor called an ambulance and Anat was rushed to the shock room, where an ultrasound showed a ruptured spleen. She had an abdominal CT scan, was given blood transfusions, and when her condition stabilized, she was hospitalized in the trauma care unit. In most cases, splenic injuries heal on their own without surgical intervention. We talked to her concerned family members and explained to them that for now she should be on a 'spleen regime' and get plenty of rest.

A few days ago, I visited Anat. She had already been hospitalized for more than two days, felt a little better and wanted to go home. At midnight I talked to the nurse in the trauma unit, and we agreed that she should have blood tests at 6 a.m. to make sure everything was okay. I got on with my work, but at the back of my mind I had a nagging feeling that she wasn't yet out of danger. At 6:30 a.m. the nurse called me, speaking rapidly, and I immediately tensed up.

"Yael, her hemoglobin is back to 6 g/cL," she told me. I had just prepared the laptop for the round after my on-call shift, and my face showed traces of a brief sleep, and for a moment I didn't know what she was talking about.

"Are you sure the blood samples aren't diluted?" I asked the nurse.

"No, we took samples twice. Come quickly."

When I arrived at the trauma unit the room was still dark and all the patients were asleep, except for Anat, who was pale and tachycardic. The nurse called the blood bank and I promptly called my on-call trauma surgeon, Dr Klein, to inform him that Anat had low hemoglobin and was hemorrhaging from the spleen.

"Come on Dreznik, this is *your* spleen," Dr Klein said. "Say goodbye to it nicely, I'll wait for you at the entrance to the OR." I breathed deeply. Meanwhile, Anat's eyes filled with tears as she spoke to her husband on the phone. I gathered the surgery consent forms and about an hour later we were in the OR to perform a splenectomy. Due to the huge amount of blood in Anat's abdomen, I knew it wouldn't be an easy procedure. I carefully grabbed the ruptured spleen and detached it from its ligaments. The sight of the severe and uncontrollable hemorrhage stressed me out and my uniform was soaked in sweat and adrenaline. We finally managed to control the bleeding and tie off the blood vessels, then I removed the spleen and handed it to the nurse with me. Dr Klein and I checked that I hadn't accidentally damaged the pancreas that is close to the spleen, and after closing the abdomen a tremendous feeling of satisfaction washed over me.

Anat seems to be recovering well and should be discharged today. She smiles at me as I check the scar her on her abdomen and I am deeply moved that this ordeal ended well.

I prepare Anat's discharge letter, then check on the rest of the patients in the trauma unit. In bed 1 lies an elderly man named Isaac, who fell off a ladder and fractured his ribs. He has since been in the trauma unit for pain relief and supervision.

Isaac smiles at me, his breathing a little heavy, a little sore. He enjoys doing odd jobs around the house and a few days ago climbed onto his roof to make repairs. Rib fractures in young people are painful but tolerable, however, in older people the condition can easily deteriorate to artificial respiration if the pain and difficulty in inflating the lungs and breathing effectively cause respiratory collapse in addition to any underlying diseases. So, we are keeping a close eye on Isaac. We examine him, and with the nurses go through his vital signs, blood gas test and last chest x-ray that shows pulmonary effusion—a buildup of fluid around the lungs.

"As far as I'm concerned, Isaac is a candidate for transfer to the internal medicine ward," Amir tells me. "Order on-call physiotherapy this evening and we'll start him on Fusid.[2] If a casualty arrives and needs a bed, Isaac will be the first to move. Update Dr Barkat from Internal ward C." We quickly go through the rest of the casualties, and I catch sight of Puta outside the trauma unit, waiting for me with a coffee. I jot down all of Amir's recommendations, give the nurses instructions, then go to the ramp for a few minutes of oxygen before the big round.

---

[2] A type of diuretic.

57

"So, what happened in the surgery with the double scrub in?" I ask Puta.

We sit on the ramp and he lights a cigarette, inhaling deeply.

"Jeez, what a letdown, I'm fed up, Dreznik. I sweated over this patient, prepared him for surgery and everything, and then doucheface comes along and takes the surgery away from me."

Doucheface is a young senior doctor who has just finished his residency with us, a douchebag who always bullied us when he was a senior resident. He's never helped in the ER and now he adds insult to injury by denying us surgeries that we wait so long for.

"I'm going to talk to the boss about this," Puta continues. "It's unacceptable, I'm not agreeing to this anymore!" I finish gulping down my coffee. I don't have anything helpful to say to Puta, all I can do is be here for him, with the 'energon cubes', and try to support him all I can during this challenging and Sisyphean residency.

My phone rings, it's Shpet.

"You want to be a pediatric surgeon, don't you?" he asks, and I could hardly contain my excitement. I remember my conversation with Miri this morning about baby Yuval, and Shay's update about an hour ago.

"Then get yourself to the OR immediately. There's a nine-month-old baby, with intussusception. Dr Shenhav is on his way, wants you to help him in the surgery. Dreznik, make me proud of you. When it's over, go straight to the ER and replace Johnny who's covering for you. Go, hurry."

3 p.m.

During my internal medicine rotation, I asked Dr Natif, our teacher, why he chose to become an internist and not, for instance, a pediatrician. He thought for a moment, then answered: "Sooner or later, you have to decide if you want to treat a patient and deal with his children, or in the case of pediatrics, deal with the parents. I'd rather deal with a patient's children than his parents." At the time, I didn't yet fully understand this rationale, but during the weeks I spent in the pediatric department and saw how taking care of a child involves taking care of an entire family, I began to grasp the complexity of being a pediatrician. Even though children may be healthier and heal better than adults, they nevertheless come with mom, dad and grandparents, which dictates the need for a different and inclusive approach for each family member, and also demands a lot of patience and tolerance.

Already back then I knew I wanted to be a pediatric surgeon. I saw it as a profession that combines surgery with society's most vulnerable members, from premature newborns to adolescents, with the opportunity to work with children of different ages and physiology and be exposed to diseases, rare tumors and birth defects. I first met Dr Shenhav, a pediatric surgeon, during my rotation in pediatric surgery, and now I am on my way to meet him again at the entrance to the OR with little baby Yuval and his parents.

Dr Shenhav takes me aside. "Dreznik, I have given the parents a detailed explanation of the surgery, but I need you to sign them on the surgery consent because I have an urgent call," he says. "Do it gently, the parents are hysterical. I trust you." Dr Shenhav is very good at "reading" parents and families. He is able to identify first time parents, sense when there are problems in the family, even if it isn't mentioned, and the moment after the parents leave his clinic, he knows if they were going to get a second opinion and who they will turn to. So, when he tells me that the parents are hysterical, he has good reason for saying it.

I look apprehensively at the parents who are sitting a few meters away from me, the father holding Yuval in his father's arms, the mother softly crying.

As I approach them the mother looks at me with suspicion and distrust. I hesitate but try to come across as confident and experienced.

"Are you Yuval Rabinovich's parents?" I ask, checking the name and sticker, and the ID band on Yuval's wrist. "Come with me," I say to the parents, "I will sign you on the surgery consent form." I begin to draw the abdomen and the stages of the surgery. "Wait a second," Ofer, the father, interrupts me. "Where is Dr Shenhav? He's going to operate, right?"

"Yes," I reply, and I will be assisting him." The father calms down, breathes a little easier, and continues to listen to me. "In the surgery we will make an incision in the lower right abdomen, similar to an incision for the removal of the appendix. Then we will gently try to clear the obstruction and see how the intestine looks, then take out the appendix." They nod, although I'm not sure that the mother is focused on what I'm saying.

"What happens if you can't clear the obstruction, if it's stuck?" the father asks, displaying a lot of worry and concern which I try to diminish and contain, aware that they will only be able to relax after the surgery.

"There are rare cases where we don't manage to clear the obstruction, or where there is bowel necrosis," I reply. "In such an event, we cut the diseased intestinal loops and perform a connection, or anastomosis, between the remaining parts." After a moment I add: "If everything goes well, you should be able to take Yuval home tomorrow afternoon." The orderly arrives and prepares the OR for surgery, the parents sign the consent form and the anesthesiologist takes baby Yuval to the OR. I escort the parents out, their eyes fixed on their son, and I tell them what I always tell parents before surgery: "I will take care of your child as if he were my own." I don't know if my words get through or bring any comfort, but they come from the heart.

"Come on, blue side and red side, get to room 1 for the evening round, " shouts Shpet in the ward corridor. Every day, including weekends, there is a big round on the entire ward with a senior surgeon, the main purpose of which is to specify and discuss the patients who are in serious general condition with impending bowel obstruction, respiratory distress, severe pancreatitis, cholecystitis, or other inflammatory state that necessitates special supervision.

On our rounds we must present a patient in a particular way, especially in a surgical round when there are more than 50 patients to get through in an hour. In medical school we were taught how to present a patient, but it can take several years to really master oral presentation skills. Just as programmers speak their own language, and military personnel have their own jargon, so doctors, everywhere in the world, have universal guidelines for conveying information, which often sounds like gibberish to a layman.

On the first day on my internal medicine rotation, Zehavit, my friend and study partner, and I were given an assignment to each choose and interview a patient, then write an admission note and present the patient to our tutor. The admission procedure consists of four stages: the medical complaint that brought the patient to the ER; the patient's medical background: diseases, medications, etc.; the overall impression of the patient following an examination; and a treatment plan. I remember being dressed in a white coat, walking around the ward and choosing to interview an elderly melanoma patient with distant metastasis, despite treatments. He had been hospitalized in the internal medicine ward for pain management and he knew his days were numbered. As I approached him, he gave me a radiant, toothless smile. He wore a shaggy hat on his head from which wisps of white hair protruded, and the sight of his emaciated body, covered with a thin blanket, was heartrending. His bed was in the corridor because all the rooms were occupied, and I sat on a chair next to him, a little in the way of the nurses briskly walking back and forth, but I didn't care.

I talked to the patient for a long time, listening to his story, completely deviating from the admission note I was assigned to write. He told me that he had three sons and had worked in construction for many years, which was evident from his rough and calloused hands. Out of the corner of my eye, I saw Zehavit talking to the patient she had chosen to interview, and like me, she was completely immersed in conversation, trying to enter her patient's world and see the illness through her eyes. Our tutor was very unimpressed with our admission notes. Zahavit's began like a novel—*Ludmila is 50 years old, married with children and works in marketing*—and didn't clearly explain why the patient was admitted, her baseline status or a treatment plan. My admission note was no less shocking; out of a hotchpotch of historical and irrelevant information, the tutor was able to extract, with difficulty, the reason for my patient's admission. However, my subsequent admission notes improved a little, and during my internship they were already much clearer, yet it was only in general surgery that I learned to write them in a purposeful, comprehensive and precise way, and I tried to explain it to the new residents who came after me, but it took them a while to learn too.

"We are operating on Yuval Rabinovitch. Intussusception reduction, no known sensitivities, *Cephamezin* before incision," I declare out loud in the OR. The monitor buzzes, Dr Shenhav hands me the scalpel. I look down at the abdomen of little Yuval, and I must work gently, precisely and with great respect. The surgery will leave a scar that he will have to live for the rest of his life and he will need to explain to others what he didn't understand at nine months old: *When I was a baby, I had an emergency surgery for an intestinal obstruction.* I make an incision, small enough for the scar to be as inconspicuous as possible, yet big enough to extract the intestine. After I get through the layer of fine muscles and the fascia, I go deep into the abdomen. We identify the caecum, a blind sac at the commencement of the large intestine, and an intestinal loop inside it, just like a telescope. The nurse hands us a wet and warm belly cloth and I gently hold the intestine, open the obstruction and pull out the small intestine. In small babies, too much force can cause a tear in the intestinal wall, because everything is so small and delicate.

While we were scrubbing in, Dr Shenhav asked me the details of the surgery, which I must have known because he lets me operate on my own and only minimally helps in the various stages of the procedure. I manage to release the small intestine and then move to the appendix, which looks slightly edematous, and perform an appendectomy. We check that everything is okay, that the intestine is normal, and then close the abdomen. I take the gentlest available Monocryl thread and suture the skin, praying that the scar will heal well. The anesthesiologist wakes up Yuval, I write a surgery report, and as Dr Shenhav and I move Yuval back to his crib, a huge smile spreads across my face. The whole procedure takes less than an hour. Outside the OR, Yuval's parents run up to me and Dr Shenhav, and on seeing my smile the mother hugs me tightly.

With Yuval's surgery behind me, I head to the ER, a long walk from the OR along an endless corridor which we have jokingly dubbed the *Walk to Canossa*.[3] My legs are starting to ache from this long day. The pager hangs on my uniform and in one pocket is the on-call phone, in the other a notepad. Suddenly and unexpectedly, my eyes fill with tears, the tears that didn't flow after this morning's terrible road accident, nor when I received chocolates from my patient at the clinic. But they are flowing now; big, warm, uncontrollable tears streaming down my face. I go into the nearest bathroom and look in the mirror. My face is red and puffy but my eyes are still shining—a clear reminder of why I chose this complex, difficult, almost impossible profession.

---

[3] An historical allusion to the arduous trek that the Roman Emperor, Henry IV, made to Pope Gregory VII at Canossa Castle in 1077.

4 p.m.

The first time I was on call in the ER, Puta accompanied me and stayed by my side for the first few hours. The awful thing about the ER is that you never know ahead of time who will walk through its doors and how you will cope. The only thing you know for certain is that your shift will eventually end. *Every shift comes to an end* is what we residents like to say. We began our shift in room 4, the triage room, while outside people flocked to the doorway, entering without permission. One patient after another came in, including a woman who got punched in the face because she made a remark to someone in a playground; a man with abdominal pain whose CT scan revealed a huge colon tumor; three girls who got out without a scratch after their car overturned, an elderly woman on blood thinners who fell and split her head open, and the list goes on. By 6 a.m., when the pressure had eased off and the triage area was relatively quiet, I too began to slow down and my heavy eyes momentarily closed while I examined a patient.

ER patients can broadly be divided into three groups: those who are discharged, those who are hospitalized, and those somewhere in the middle, the most challenging patients for whom we can't pinpoint a diagnosis. Do they have a problem that requires surgery? Do they have an internal problem that we can't get to the bottom of? We must be able to make a decision, taking into account that it might be a wrong decision.

Over time, we residents have established some sacred rules that we follow. One of them is the 'surgical spirit' rule, according to which surgeons go the extra mile for patients in their care, or formerly in their care, without turning their back on them. For instance, when patients who we operated on in the past return to the ER full of metastasis and needs pain relief or a morphine drip, we extend our care to them and admit them with us rather than transfer them to the internal medicine ward. However, Shpet sometimes gets angry that our 'surgical spirit' is not in line with other surgical specialties.

Another sacred rule determines that if the ER is not swamped by midnight, the shift will go well. This rule has two exceptions, namely the 'two big jokers' that can turn the ER into a surgical war zone by 4 a.m. The first joker is multi-trauma, such as a serious car accident with multiple victims or injuries, which trumps all the cards. The second joker is a patient with an acute intestinal ischemia, for instance, mesenteric ischemia—as in the case of our Shoshana who is currently in intensive care—and for some reason these patients tend to come to the ER early in the morning. One of our senior doctors once joked that they probably wait quietly behind the bushes outside the ER and emerge just as a resident decides to take forty winks at around 5 a.m. Besides these 'two big jokers', it isn't uncommon for our pager to beep with other surprises—some of which are very peculiar—just before we sink into a broken sleep on a bug-infested mattress. I'll never forget, for instance, the case of a schizophrenic patient who was sure there was a huge worm hiding in her rectum, which she decided to remove with pliers, and in doing so perforated her anus.

Back at the ER, I meet Johnny in room 4. He's on the computer and smiles at me.

"Dreznik, there are two patients for the time being: an elderly woman named Osnat with abdominal pain, her second referral to the ER...the story's not clear. And a 45-year-old jaundiced patient, Aviad, with a high level of bilirubin—above 10mg in lab tests. First of all, close all their details and then be available for all the sutures and the other patients waiting for you. I'm going to the OR, Shpet and I are about to go into surgery—an appendectomy—then we'll come and help you."

Johnny is a good friend who always seems to appear when I need him most. Two weeks earlier on a Sunday, Johnny and I were on call together. I did a good deed and replaced a resident who had to attend a wedding that day, and hoped I would be rewarded for my act of kindness with an easy shift. Puta chuckled maliciously, smiling his rascally smile, assuring me that it was going to be a horrible day, because Sundays always are. We more or less know what to expect in the ER each day of the week. Sunday is the worst day when a lot of patients are registered in the ER, some of them in very serious condition. Monday through Thursday the work is steady, but it changes from time to time. Friday usually started out busy with many people coming in before the weekend, and gradually quietens down by nightfall. Saturday is the opposite, starting out relatively quiet and ending up like Grand Central Station.

On that particular Sunday, I arrived at the ER, not looking forward to the prospect of carrying the weight of the world on my shoulders. I breathed a momentary sigh of relief when I saw only six patients on the dashboard; maybe the 'man upstairs' was answering my prayers after all. However, not twenty minutes had passed, and as luck would have it, lots of people came streaming in, as if a bus had stopped outside and unloaded all the stomachaches that had been waiting all weekend to come to the ER that day at precisely 4 p.m. Johnny and another senior resident went to the OR for two appendectomies, while I ran around like a headless chicken, trying to juggle a construction worker who had fallen from a building, an elderly woman writhing in agony, and an elderly man with a high fever. At my most difficult moment Johnny suddenly appeared like an angel from heaven and said his well-known phrase: *A French prostitute can't give more than she has, and if she doesn't have enough—she brings her sister along.*

It's now 4:20 p.m. and the first patient I see in the ER is Osnat, who, according to the computer is a retired 68-years old widow and an active grandmother. The triage nurse has taken her vital signs, and although she's a little tachycardic, her blood pressure is normal and she has no fever. She came to the ER two days ago complaining of abdominal pain and since her lab tests and abdominal x-ray were normal, she was discharged and told to follow-up with her family doctor. The nurse's report is brief— abdominal pain and swelling, second visit to the ER, no vomiting—yet contained enough information for me to dig deeper into my investigation. Most ERs around the world have a policy regarding the return of patients within a week, which is usually determined by a health authority that has established a specific procedure that goes along these lines:

A return visit to the ER within a short time can indicate a need to reassess the diagnosis and treatment established in the previous visit, and therefore special consideration and extra caution is required when making diagnostic and treatment decisions.

Osnat walks heavily to a chair opposite me and sits down with her two grownup daughters who accompany her. She looks at me with hopeful eyes and asks me the cause of her severe pain, which began a few days earlier.

"My belly is swollen," she says, pointing to a slightly swollen abdomen. "I feel like I've gained weight in the last few days." I exchange a few words with her, ask her about illnesses, medications she has taken, if she has undergone any surgeries. She tells me she has never suffered from a significant medical problem. She climbs onto the examination bed with difficulty; she clearly has no rest from her pain, and on examination I do not feel a lump in her abdomen or any signs of considerable sensitivity. Her blood tests are back and they too seem normal. Yet I am still concerned. I speak to the on-call radiologist, present the case to him, and manage to convince him to do an abdominal CT scan, insisting that it must be done now through the emergency department so that we can get an immediate answer. I explain to Osnat that she will have to drink a CT contrast material and that hopefully we will have a diagnosis in about two hours.

Just before I call my next patient, I leave the room, following Osnat with my eyes, and see a smiling couple sitting on the bench waiting for me. I recognize Aviad with the jaundice who Johnny told me about. "Hi, doctor," Aviad's wife, Dana, cheerfully greets me. "When do you think we'll be able to go home?" Aviad smiles at her, and I can't help but smile at her too.

A few minutes later they are sitting in my room, after I have looked over the results of Aviad's blood tests and read a letter of referral from his family doctor: *Forty-five years old, generally healthy, married and father of three. In the last few days, signs of jaundice in addition to itching. No fever, no vomiting or diarrhea. No weight loss. He had an ultrasound that showed a little sediment in the gallbladder. Due to worsening jaundice, I am referring him to the ER for further investigation."*

Dana tells me they have three children, that she is a teacher and Aviad works at an insurance company and is in good health. His mother had a cholecystectomy—could that be related? I look at the results of the ultrasound Aviad brought with him, then I examine him but don't feel anything suspicious.

"I think you should be hospitalized in order to continue the investigation," I say. "First we'll do another ultrasound," I add. Dana frowns at me, clearly not taking kindly to my advice.

Patients have mixed feelings about being admitted. On the one hand, no one enjoys being hospitalized; it's not something that anyone plans for. On the other hand, it brings some relief from their helpless suffering at home from a condition for which there is no home remedy or medication. I listen to Aviad, who doesn't want to be hospitalized, then take a piece of paper and start drawing.

"Look, this is the gallbladder," I explain. "Chances are a stone in your gallbladder has migrated into the common bile duct and caused jaundice. Sometimes the gallstone remains stuck there and needs to be removed endoscopically. It could be that the jaundice is due to other reasons, but in any case, I can't let you go home," I conclude. And even though I am running behind schedule and the dashboard is filling up with more patients, we talk a little more. It's strange, but Aviad and Dana recharge me with energy; there is some kind of chemistry between us that is hard to explain, and as they get up to leave, Dana promises to bring me a coffee from the cafeteria.

5 p.m.

I finish arranging hospitalization for Aviad and the CT forms for Osnat and go to the triage area. Johnny and Shpet are in surgery, and I am now responsible for everything that occurs in the ER, the mess in the trauma unit, and of course the ward, which is currently being managed by two interns. Sometimes this responsibility is inconceivable, especially when several difficult cases arise simultaneously, and I have to prioritize the order of patient care within seconds. My phone beeps, it's Gadi texting me that he is on his way home to release the nanny and take care of the girls, and I remember being off duty last weekend and enjoying time at home with my family.

Residency varies from days when I don't see my family, to days when I have time on my hands. I take the girls to a café, tidy the house, watch a movie with Gadi or occasionally go on a day trip. This past weekend was just like that. It was a warm Saturday and we all went to the National Park, which I remember from my childhood, back when it had a lakeside restaurant and colorful rowboats. My friends and I had a picnic there after graduation, and years later I took Tamar and we went on a train ride round the park. Even though there's always a long stretch of time between visits to the park, the trees never seem to change over time, and the train, its colors now a little faded, looks exactly the same, as does the lake water, only without the row boats.

The girls and I were on the swings, soaring high, observing the tall trees at the end of the park. I had quiet thoughts about the meaning of life, the kind of thoughts that don't usually cross my mind, not even when I inform patients that they are terminally ill, because my head is constantly preoccupied with the next task for fear of getting emotionally immersed in the devastating news. But that Saturday on the swing, I allowed myself to get lost in thought. I looked at the girls swaying in the wind and giggling their thoughts out loud, and I wanted to imagine when I would be here again,

69

what I would still have to go through, and how many more patients would leave a scar on my heart.

"Do you want us to drop by and visit you at the hospital?" Gadi texts me. From time to time, Gadi and the girls surprise me and drop by the hospital with food, which warms my heart and boosts my energy for the rest of the shift. "There's no need," I text back, "it's been a difficult day so far, and I still don't know how the rest of it will pan out." I see Erez, the nurse in charge of the ER, in the triage area and he asks me if it's quiet.

"Erez, some things need to go unsaid," I reply, and he chuckles. If there is one thing that should never be said in the ER, it is any kind of reference to how quiet it is or how smoothly things are running, and when someone does say the unsaid, through a slip of the tongue, everyone around knocks on wood so as not to tempt fate. In a life of unknowns and uncertainty, superstitions are sometimes the only thing that keeps us sane.

I go to the treatment room where an elderly woman who fell and cut open her forehead is lying on a bed, patiently waiting for me to suture her deep wound. I don sterile gloves and apply lidocaine, a local anesthesia, to her forehead. Meanwhile, the nurses in the trauma unit are monitoring Isaac, who fell of a ladder and broke several ribs. He looks worse than he did at noon, his breathing now quick and heavy, and the saturation that measures the oxygen in his blood is starting to drop. The nurses connect him to an oxygen enrichment mask, add an inhaler and another pain reliever. But not long after I finish suturing, I get a call from the trauma unit, and I know what it's about. "Come quickly, Isaac is in bed 1, he doesn't look well."

I remove my gloves and leave the commotion in the ER, including at least five people in the admission process waiting for me to examine them, all glaring at me as I walk away. And who knows how many more patients there are in the triage area in critical condition and in need of surgery. As I quickly climb the stairs to the trauma unit, I call my attending trauma surgeon, Amir. We are taught not to bother the senior doctors until we formulate a work plan, which involves first examining the patient, taking lab tests and formulating a solution that includes the relevant imaging and specific consultation. So, my conversation with Dr Amir would go something like this: *A patient in room 1 worries me. He is breathing over thirty breaths per minute, he has low blood pressure, his oxygen saturation level is about 90%, and the blood gases I just took indicate an accumulation of carbon dioxide. I think he should be connected to a BiPAP machine, and I'm considering intubation.*

However, in Isaac's case, I have a bad gut feeling, one that tells me I don't have time to prepare an orderly treatment plan before the senior arrives. Amir answers my call immediately, and we meet at the entrance to the trauma unit, where Isaac's son is waiting, clearly very concerned.

"I spoke to my dad a few minutes ago," he says, "and suddenly he stopped responding to me, I don't know what happened to him." I look at Isaac, who smiled at me a few hours ago, and apart from a few broken ribs he had no medical problems. But now his monitor is going completely crazy, and I watch as he suddenly rolls his eyes and collapses.

"CPR *now*," Amir calls out with restraint, but loud enough for the staff in the room to hear and move into a completely different operating model. If I had had time in those seconds to think about the mechanism—such as a pulmonary embolism that results from prolonged lying down and lack of movement, which in turn can lead to arrhythmias and ventricular fibrillation—I would have, but at this critical moment I am in emergency mode. Unlike the chaos of the shock room, the chaos created during CPR follows a particular order: A senior doctor is in charge of the CPR management and decides when the cycles of chest compressions change, when to give adrenaline, when to attach the defibrillator to the patient, and so forth. Someone else is responsible for the Ambu[4] and intubation, at least two others perform the cycles of compressions, and another person administers medical treatment, such as adrenaline, dobutamine and magnesium. We remove all the family members from the trauma unit and get to work

---

[4] A manual resuscitator.

on Isaac. I can't feel his pulse and realize that we are running out of time and must act quickly so as to conserve the remaining oxygen in his body.

Compressions are extremely difficult to do. I need to do thirty, forcefully, into Isaac's chest. I feel the muscles of my hands and arms stretching and hear myself count aloud—*twenty-four, twenty-five, twenty-six*, and I see Latif, the nurse next to me, preparing to replace me. We are on another round of intravenous adrenaline and we stop for a second to check if the pulse has returned, but to no avail. We continue. Amir dictates the rhythm and I lose all sense of time, which seems like an eternity. in CPR there is always the question of when to stop. Some studies indicate that after half an hour of CPR irreversible brain damage has already occurred, but there are case studies that report of miracles and people who fully recover after prolonged CPR.

We fight for Isaac, but his pulse doesn't return and there are no signs of it returning. I suddenly hear Amir's voice, as if in a dream, telling us to stop.

"Guys, we've been doing CPR for over 40 minutes, let's do a situation assessment," he says, and I know that now he will make the most difficult decision in CPR: the decision to stop. "Time of death 5:50 p.m., Amir says in a cracked voice. "Dreznik, do an ECG and fill out the forms, I'll talk to the family. May his memory be blessed." I look at Amir, who was with me this morning in the shock room when we lost the young woman. This is our second death in one day. We are never really prepared for the death of a patient, not even a terminal patient on a morphine drip, whose heart monitor can flatline at any moment, leaving another scar on our hearts. Over time most of the scars fade but there are some that never completely heal.

"What's up Dreznik? We've finished the appendectomy and are coming to help you in the ER," Shpet mumbles to me through his phone. As I collapse into a chair, he hears me let out a long sigh, then the trembling in my voice as tears well up in my eyes. I start to tell him about Isaac and the long CPR and what still awaits me in the ER, but he interrupts my flow of words: "Let's meet at the fish pond near the ER. Me, you and

Johnny will share the tasks. And Dreznik..." he pauses, "it's a tough day, and you're getting through it big time. It may be a difficult shift, but we'll beat it."

6 p.m.

I contemplate the next twelve hours before Puta and Imrish arrive for the morning round. I'm now half way through my shift, the minutes and hours intertwined with all the things I've done so far, like a puzzle made up of a million people I've seen, all mixed up in my head. I finish up in the trauma unit. After the chaos of the CPR and Isaac's sudden departure from the world, a heavy silence pervades the room. The nurses remove the electrodes from Isaac's chest and clean him, and the auxiliary staff thoroughly disinfect the area. Soon the paramedics will remove Isaac from the trauma unit and the funeral arrangements will begin. I finish doing an ECG that shows a flatline…I so hate this moment.

During medical school, I had the opportunity to study at the National Center of Forensic Medicine in Tel Aviv. There is something about the finality of death that has fascinated me since I began studying medicine; the notion that one moment we are an entire world, and the next we are corpses laid out on shiny iron beds. And I have always wondered where we disappear to after death. The question of the afterlife has intrigued humanity since time immemorial, so it's little wonder there are so many theories about the immortality of the soul and numerous explanations for a concept that we are not really able to grasp and digest. On my first day at the Center, I met the head, a well-known professor at the morgue, and watched him closely examine a little three-month-old baby lying on an iron bed. I couldn't understand why the baby wasn't crying, and a long minute passed before I realized that the baby was dead. I recall this day in great detail, the feeling that everything around me was happening in slow-motion and I was observing myself from outside my body.

An autopsy, is a step-by-step procedure that begins with an external examination and everything seen on the body is recorded. We once examined a street prostitute who was found dead on the sidewalk, and our recording went as follows: *Patient about forty years old, an eagle-type tattoo on her right shoulder, two fentanyl patches on her back, a longitudinal scar on her left arm.*

The next stage is the autopsy prosection—the dissection of the cadaver. The skin of the scalp is removed and the brain is exposed, then a longitudinal incision is made from the neck almost to the pelvis and all the internal organs are removed: heart, stomach, large intestine, small intestine, lungs, liver and so forth, which are checked for any indications of a violent or unnatural death. Once we found a hematoma on the muscles in the frontal part of the neck—the infrahyoid muscles—which raised suspicion of suffocation. Another time, we saw gunpowder close to the temple, which indicated suicide by a close-range gunshot. Once the prosection is completed, a detailed forensic report is written up.

Lunch at the National Center of Forensic Medicine was a huge and varied buffet, and to this day I remember the smell of potatoes cooked in garlic and olive oil. On my first day there I couldn't eat anything, but my appetite quickly returned. Every time I left the center at the end of a long day of examining cadavers, it was like coming out of the valley of death, and my return to the world outside seemed like a vague dream.

Every time I determine a death on the ward and attach the ECG stickers to the chest of my deceased patient, I again felt the coldness of death around me, enveloping me and not letting go until I leave the room and wash my hands and heart. Just as I feel now as I say goodbye to Isaac and sign on the flatline of the ECG. There are some things in life that we are never able to fully grasp and come to terms with.

The ER dashboard looks like a war zone. Just before I go down to the fish pond to meet Johnny and Shpet, I count at least 20 patients marked in red. There are about 10 patients in the ER, next to room 4 and the triage—these are usually the least urgent—and the same number in the large ER, with no end in sight. We have our work cut out for us.

Johnny, Shpet and I only have a few minutes to exchange information. Thankfully Johnny brings a large bag of potato chips from the vending machine; it's been a few hours since I ate my sandwich and my stomach is empty again. The three of us sit by the fish pond and dive into the potato chips, our fingers greasy and salty, while Shpet gives us a rundown of our tasks.

"Listen carefully," he begins, "I'm going to the ward to see all the asterisks. Johnny, there's someone in triage with an intestinal obstruction I want you to see, Frankel I think his name is, and later there's a consult on Internal Ward B. Dreznik, quickly get the triage unit under control, then go to the other patients in the large ER."

I tell them about the CPR. It's likely that we'll present Isaac's case at our next M&M[5] meeting and try to draw conclusions from this unexpected death. Shpet polishes off the rest of the potato chips then pulls out a cold can of cola from his pocket.

"Take it, Dreznik," he says, handing me the can. Then we split up, each going his own way until our paths cross again. I gulp down the cola with bits of chewed potato chips, but it's the most comforting drink I've had all day.

In the triage I catch a glance of Osnat, the patient with abdominal pain who has finished drinking the contrast material and is about to do a CT scan. There are also several patients waiting to see me, including a young woman who looks like she's recently given birth. Varda, the nurse who works with me in the triage, informs me that the young woman is in a lot of pain, has a fever, and is showing signs of mastitis.[6] I look at her and suddenly have a flashback of my own first postpartum experience. As I approach her, I sense relief in her eyes, perhaps because I'm a female doctor. I take her into the room.

"Noga, right?" She sits down, I turn on the computer again and take her details and medical history. "So Noga, is this your first birth?" I ask. She nods and tears roll down her cheeks. Her phone rings and she quickly answers it.

"Yes, I'm with the surgeon, give her a bottle in the meantime," she says and hangs up. The sight of Noga throws me back several years to the anxiety that consumed

---

[5] Morbidity & Mortality
[6] Breast infection

me after giving birth, the fluctuating hormones, the burning pain from breastfeeding, the episiotomy incision and stitches. I sense that Noga feels very alone right now and I want to comfort her. She tells me that in the last few days she has been in agonizing pain from breastfeeding.

"My baby wants to eat, but breastfeeding her is so painful...I can't take it anymore. And yesterday I developed a fever and now my breast is sensitive and painful and red." I feel her pain, as though it was me sitting there. Before I examine her, I ask her if she has any medical problems, past illnesses, drug intolerance, and what she named her baby. Noga smiles through her tears.

"Her name is Yael, like you," she says, and I smile back. I ask her to lie on the treatment bed, but just then the radiologist calls me.

"You should come see the CT scan of Osnat with the abdominal pain," he says. I apologize to Noga, promising to return in a few minutes.

7 p.m.

In medical school we had a course on how to break bad news to a patient, and at the time it seemed easy. A psychologist explained to us the protocol: how to break the news and to whom, what to say and what not to say; what to do when a patient doesn't want to hear everything; what to do when the family doesn't want the patient to know his or her diagnosis, and so forth. Then we did simulation training, with actors trained to simulate real patients, and we had to inform them that they were seriously ill with a disease that was written on a piece of paper we were handed on our way into the simulation room. The actors largely improvised, changing their behavior and response to the bad news in each simulation, so that we too had to improvise our way through the conversation and deal with it as best we could.

In one of my simulations, when I told a 'patient' that she had multiple sclerosis, she began crying and shouting, but I managed to calm her down, and in the end we shook hands and politely parted. Most of our simulations were in our final year of medical school during the month of June, by which time we were largely preoccupied with summer plans, eager to hit the beach, soak up the sun. So, we didn't take all the talk about diseases and bad new too seriously or consider it relevant to our lives.

Fast forward four years. It's now 7:15 p.m. and I am thinking about Osnat, a lovely 68-year-old woman with soft blue eyes, and how for several days she has had a swollen abdomen accompanied by a nagging pain.

Two weeks ago, we celebrated Rosh Hashana. I have a custom that at the beginning of every new year I write three wishes on a piece of and place it under my pillow for safekeeping. I wish one thing for myself and two for my family. I began this custom when I was 18 and terribly depressed because I had just failed my driving test. Out of desperation I wrote a note wishing for a more successful year, to find a boyfriend and to get a driver's license. These wishes materialized, and since then I have kept up this custom as an integral part of the new year.

Osnat's CT scan shows that her entire abdomen is lined with a tumor and lumps of tumor tissue that envelop the intestines and the abdominal cavity. In the past we had such a patient on the ward, who was wasting away before our eyes, and we had him transferred to oncology where he started chemotherapy. This is often an aggressive tumor, whose source cannot always be determined, and it spreads in the abdomen causing ascites that keeps accumulating. Chemotherapy helps very little, if at all. I look at Osnat's CT scan and think of the piece of paper under my pillow, realizing that at some stage in life we are all paper-thin, blowing in the wind. I see Osnat's daughters in the distance. They know that their mother has already had the CT scan, and apparently the results are through, so I try not to meet their eyes. Always before delivering bad news, my stomach churns and I find myself taking deep breaths, as if preparing myself before jumping into a deep pool of cold water. I feel as though someone has placed weights on my shoulders and I am helplessly sinking. And the truth is, it never really gets easier with time. I try to find the right words to say, aware of the subtleties that every patient needs. I shall never forget the first patient to whom I delivered bad news—Mrs Laor.

One evening, barely a month into my residency, while driving home from the hospital, the thought of Mrs Laor weighed heavy on my heart and I couldn't erase the image of her eyes from my mind. Even the girls' little giggles in bed couldn't alleviate my sadness. Mrs Laor was a tiny woman of about 70, widowed for many years, with a partner who took care of her and never left her side. She had come to the ER with vomitus that looked a little black. We performed a gastroscopy, which looked normal and sent her home. A few days later I saw her again on the ward; she was having again multiple vomiting episodes. An x-ray showed a huge stomach, and it was clear that there was some kind of gastric outlet obstruction. I anxiously waited for the CT scan to see what was causing the vomiting, and I remember that as soon as I saw the scan, I understood the problem. Mrs Laor had a huge tumor in the retroperitoneum which blocked almost the entire third part of the duodenum, and the metastases had probably reached the lungs and bones. That same day was the first time that I delivered tragic news to a patient. I approached her bed and told her and her partner that she had a tumor that was pressing on the stomach and the duodenum, and that we planned to take a biopsy. I was careful not to mention the metastases, nor did I tell her that the tumor was almost certainly malignant. I desperately hoped that it was a lymphoma that could be shrunk with chemotherapy, and rushed Mrs Laor to gastric bypass surgery combined with a biopsy so that she could eat. But within a few days the result came back that it was metastatic adenocarcinoma, and even the oncologist had nothing comforting to say, because there really was no treatment for this type of cancer.

I went to visit Mrs Laor again. My steps were heavy and the way to her room was long and tense. I felt like the messenger in the *Book of Job*, who came to bear Job bad news. Her partner was not in the room with her, and despite looking for him, he was nowhere to be found. Mrs Laor was sitting up in bed, talking to one of her children on the phone, and her eyes met mine. I sat down in a chair next to her, and she asked me if the results of the biopsy had come through. I looked down. What a hard-to-swallow moment. "It's adenocarcinoma," I finally managed to say, and she holds her breath for a second. Then she shared with me that she had nothing to fight for. She told how her husband deteriorated and began to shut down after he started cancer treatment, lying in the hospital bed with diapers, staring into space. As she spoke her eyes began to water and a tear fell from mine. I reached out and held her hand, and her bright blue eyes stared into mine.

"You knew all along, didn't you?" she said suddenly. "You felt it." And as I left her room, I cursed this profession for the first time in my life.

"Noga?" I call again to the young woman sitting outside. I have just finished talking with Osnat, who left the room with her daughters supporting her, because after hearing her diagnosis, her legs almost gave out. The room closes in on me, like it did with Mrs Laor. I can't breathe. Patients always remember the moment they are given bad news, when their lives turn upside down. They always remember our words: *Look, we see some indeterminate lump on your CT which we need to characterize and see how we are going to take a biopsy, but that explains your pain.* and then the world converges on the subtleties of the tone of speech and the ensuing silence. The hopelessness of it all burns a hole in my heart that only I can feel. And although I know that it will heal with time, right now the hole is so tangible and huge that I'm just waiting to fill it in my conversation with Noga.

I proceed to examine her. While palpating the left breast I feel significant inflammation, it is swollen red and sensitive, maybe there is even an abscess. Noga is suffering, she's in pain, and I ask her to wait a second while I bring the ultrasound device from the treatment room. I place the probe on the swollen, red breast and see a large cavity that looks like an abscess. A large part of our work is draining abscesses that can form in different parts in the body, including the breast, where an abscess can form as a result of mastitis. Draining a breast abscess is a very delicate procedure; it is better to suck out the fluid with a needle rather than cut the abscess open with a scalpel, so as not to damage the tissue of the breast ducts. Drainage is necessary because there is little to no chance that antibiotics alone will work. I tell Noga that I am going to drain the cavity of pus with a needle, that it will hurt a little and after the procedure she will need to be admitted. I don sterile gloves, take a pad dipped in alcohol and a pink needle for suction, and ask Noga to lie still with her arms raised. She is tense and nervous, afraid of the prick, but keeps perfectly still as I disinfect the area, and with the ultrasound guiding me I suck out about 20 cc of purulent fluid from the breast. I explain to Noga that the pus pocket has shrunk, but may fill up again in the next day or two, so she will need intravenous antibiotic therapy and a follow-up ultrasound. I tell her what to expect next and reassure her that everything will be fine, which I was unable to do in Osnat's case. I imagine for a second what it would be like if all diseases were mere abscesses that could be drained from the body.

My phone rings, it's Johnny, calling from the triage area. "Dreznik," he begins, "there's a Mr Frankel here with an intestinal obstruction. Let's hospitalize him and try to treat him conservatively with a nasogastric tube. Just know that he's here. I'm going to Internal Ward B, someone there has bleeding hemorrhoids. It's quite serious, so you'll be on your own now. There's also someone here by the name of Shaked, a 70-something-year-old man whose abdominal CT scan shows he has diverticulitis.[7] Just check on him to see that he's in reasonable condition and schedule him for hospitalization with Shpet."

I once again abandon the triage unit, where casualties from two minor car accidents await me, and head to the large ER area, taking the opportunity to drink a cup of water on the way and trying to remember why the name Shaked rings a bell.

As I log in to the computer in the triage area, I suddenly remember that I met Mr Shaked on my previous shift. He came to the ER with his wife, complaining of slight pain in the lower left abdomen. We found nothing unusual and the lab tests were all fine except for a small increase in white blood cells. I took a look at the discharge letter I wrote: *75 years old with a background of hypertension. Lower left abdominal pain for two days, no vomiting, no diarrhea, no fever. On examination minimal sensitivity in the lower abdomen; Lab tests show mild leukocytosis. In conclusion, no current evidence of an acute surgical problem. Follow-up with a family doctor is recommended and if the condition worsens, please return to the ER. A colonoscopy should be carried out as per the recommendations.* I feel my heart rate increase slightly. This is a patient who, a few days ago, I sent home, and it turns out he had a problem that I failed to diagnose, and now he's back with significantly more inflammation. I quickly open the CT scan that he did in the ER, and see severe inflammation of the left colon caused by diverticulitis, a common disease among the elderly. This is usually treated with antibiotics, and it's possible that had I correctly diagnosed the patient a few days ago and prescribed antibiotics, or investigated further, he wouldn't be in the ER now in a worse condition. I have a feeling that Johnny was aware of this, but didn't want to tell me explicitly that I

---

[7] Inflammation of pouches in the colon wall.

had messed up, since the damage had probably already been done. I head to Mr Shaked's room, hoping to God I get out of there in one piece.

8 p.m.

On the way I pass one of the nurses from the ER who tells me that the patient Shaked looks more like Sha*dead*, which only exacerbates my anxiety. When I was little, my parents used to tell me: *Yael, it's only those who do nothing that make no mistakes*, but you can't compare a mistake made by an economist, for instance, to a mistake made by a doctor, which can be a matter of life or death. In medicine, all kinds of mistakes can be made, such as administering the wrong dose of medication, that can be fatal. There are also mistakes that result from a lack of knowledge, medical negligence, system overload or not noticing the signs or red lights vis á vis a patient. The French surgeon, Rene Leriche, once said: "Every surgeon carries within him a small cemetery, where from time to time he goes to pray – a place of bitterness and regret, where he must look for an explanation for his failures." As surgeons, we are aware of this aphorism the day we qualify as doctors and take the physician's oath, but I'm not sure that we can actually live with this painful fact without repressing it deep inside us.

I approach cubicle 9 in the ER. I recognize Shaked, a nice man, retired. He is lying in bed, looking a little paler than when I saw him last. His wife, a petite, hunchbacked lady, is sitting next to him, looking at me with curiosity, then a flash of recognition appears on her face.

"You're the doctor who met us a few days ago, the one who let him go home," she remarks. I nod, smile and remain silent, lost for words. *It's only those who do nothing that make no mistakes*, echoes in my head, as I shake Shaked's hand, and he nods, with no blame or doubt in his eyes. He mostly wants an answer to his pain, wants to know what will happen now. I examine him and there is tenderness in the lower left abdomen, but to my relief he has no signs of peritonitis and the diverticulitis can be treated with antibiotics and hospitalization.

I explain to Shaked and his wife what diverticulitis is, make a sketch of the colon, explain that over the years pouches—small protrusions of tissue—similar to hernias form in the colon. These pouches can cause several problems, one of which is bleeding. The second problem is inflammation, which Mr Shaked has. The inflammation can be simple or it can be complex with formation of a hole in the pouch and a breakthrough of feces from the large intestine into the abdominal cavity - a life-threatening situation. They listen to my explanation, and I immediately reassure them that according to the CT scan, the inflammation does not appear to be significant, but that it does require hospitalization and intravenous antibiotics, and that I believe everything will be fine. They don't ask me why I discharged them a few days ago without any treatment. They may be wondering why, and will perhaps tell their family how the doctor was wrong the first time, and how lucky that it was caught in time. They may praise the doctor who insisted on doing a CT-scan today in the ER, but that's out of my hands. The doctor who persists in finding the correct diagnoses, after several wrong diagnoses, is always the one who's right; that's how it is, how it's always been, and how it always will be, everywhere in the world. It's like the abdominal CT scan I insisted on for Osnat with the diffuse intra-abdominal tumor, who, despite falling into a bottomless pit, looked at me as if to say: *She's the one who diagnosed me, she got it right, she's a good doctor.* I gather my strength to continue the shift, say goodbye to the Shakeds, write up the follow-up on the computer and inform the interns on the ward of Mr Shaked's hospitalization. Then in the small notebook I carry with me everywhere, I write Shaked's name; this is my way of trying to learn from my mistakes, or at least not to repeat them.

On my way to the bathroom, I glance at the clock. Time is passing quickly, it's almost 9 p.m. I finish seeing two young men who were in a minor rear-end collision, one of whom has neck pain. On almost every shift in the ER several minor casualties from car accidents come in and take up a lot of time, energy and excessive paperwork when all they have is a whiplash injury due to a sudden jerk of the head in a forward or backward motion, causing slight sensitivity and stiffness of the neck muscles. Witnesses to the road accident, and often the police, recommend going to the ER, mainly because of the insurance or due to lack of knowledge. So, half of my time in the triage unit is taken up with whiplash casualties, basically telling them they'll be fine and sending them home. Other than that, there isn't much I can do for them medically.

Shpet receives a call from Johnny, who is still on Internal Ward B in the room of Mr Sa'adi, a dialysis patient whose hemorrhoids are bleeding. There are blood stains on the sheet, a puddle of blood on the floor and Mr Sa'adi's diaper is soaked in blood. The room looks like a slaughterhouse.

"Is he hemodynamically stable?" Shpet asks Johnny.

"His blood pressure is fine in the meantime…he's been suffering from hemorrhoids for years," Johnny replies. "Today he had dialysis and for about two hours now the bleeding keeps coming back," he adds, then informs the nurse and the internist that Mr Sa'adi will move to our ward for close surveillance and perhaps an urgent hemorrhoidectomy.

"All right," says Shpet, "make sure he gets to our ward quickly and put him in a room near the nurses' station. Get Gelfoam from the OR and as soon as he arrives, have Dreznik insert a femoral central line. I've just been on the ward, it's quiet. I'm going back to the ER to see patients."

During our shifts we are responsible for the general surgical ward, the trauma unit and the ER department. However, in practice, every patient in the hospital can suffer from a surgical problem that requires surgical consultation and assessment. For instance, we are often called to the maternity ward to repair a perineal tear that was caused during childbirth and which requires special suturing, or to the pediatric surgery department where there are patients we need to examine.

Johnny updates me on the new admissions, and just as I'm telling him about Shaked, I suddenly see a familiar face at the entrance to the ER. I tax my tired brain trying to remember who it is, and suddenly the penny drops.

"Alon Zinger!" I call out. He turns his gaze to me, with a wide, coy smile.

"Dreznik, what are you doing here?" He is dressed in a suit and an attractive blonde woman is sitting next to him, looking tense. Alon introduces her to me.

"This is Yael, she studied economics with me."

I shake their hands, remembering days gone by—days of economics and the Ministry of Finance. It seems so long ago.

"What are *you* doing here?" I inquire, realizing that he needs a surgeon and hope that it's not a serious problem.

"I'm ashamed to tell you," Alon replies, stammering a little, "but we were playing with a love egg and it got stuck." He blushes.

"Stuck where?" I ask, but already know the answer.

"I put it up my...you know... rectum, and I can't get it out. My wife doesn't know anything. I'm so glad you're here...you've got to help me..."

Alon and I studied together for undergraduate and postgraduate degrees in economics, and passed our final exams by the skin of our teeth. I got accepted to the Ministry of Finance, and Alon applied for a job at an investment company. I last saw him in my mid-20s when I was heavily pregnant with Tamar, before changing my career path to medicine.

It was late evening. From the window of my office in Jerusalem, I admired the hills and felt the evening chill of Jerusalem come in through the open window. I was in the capital market department on the fifth floor of the Ministry of Finance building, decorated with climbing plants. Despite my advanced pregnancy and an hour's drive home, I needed to stay late at the office to rewrite a draft of new reform regulations for the Finance Committee. Suddenly, out of the corner of my eye, I saw Alon, who had arrived for a meeting with my boss. Although our friendship had dwindled a little, we still kept in touch, so I was very happy to see him. He wore a white shirt and tie, shiny shoes and held a black briefcase. He approached me with an animated smile. "Dreznik, what's going on? How's the treasury? Working hard?" We chatted for a while and he told me about his work in the private sector. Who would have thought that our paths would meet again in the ER years later in such embarrassing circumstances?

Johnny rings me again."Dreznik, get ready to come to the ward in half an hour. A nice man called Sa'adi is coming to us from the internal ward with bleeding hemorrhoids. Shpet wants you to insert a femoral venous line and we'll start giving him blood." I end the call and look at Alon Zinger, who looks back at me with questioning eyes.

"Listen," I say, "I'll fill out a form for you for an abdominal x-ray. If the egg is deep in the rectum, we'll have to remove it like in a colonoscopy examination. If it's close to the anus, we'll try another option."

"I have to go home today," he says. "I have no idea how I got myself into this mess." I discern deep concern in his eyes and promise to try and help him as soon as possible.

9 p.m.

After the ER has calmed down a little, I go up to the ward, thinking about Alon Zinger, about the egg stuck in his butthole and let out a stifled laugh, eager to relate the juicy story to Shpet and Johnny. We have a whole collection of bizarre and peculiar stories, testifying to the complexity of the human race, stories that you don't hear about in other workplaces. Alon's story reminds me of Shiri, a 16-year-old girl I met about two months ago, during my rotation in pediatric surgery.

Shiri was an 11th grade student, a quiet introverted girl. She came to the ER with abdominal pain that had intensified. I saw her for the first time in the pediatric ER, examined her and sent her for an abdominal x-ray, which showed a huge, enlarged stomach with a mass of something that we were unable to identify. From there Shiri did a gastroscopy, which revealed a clump of hair stuck in her stomach that couldn't be removed. In our psychiatric course at medical school, we learned about a psychiatric disorder known as Rapunzel syndrome, a rare disorder that manifests itself by pulling out hairs—mostly scalp hairs— then chewing and swallowing them. The problem is that hairs are not digested in the digestive system and over time they become a plug of hair that gets stuck in the stomach, causing a blockage. After the gastroscopy, I talked to Shiri's parents, who were shocked at the whole thing, and when Shiri woke up, I asked her if she pulled out hairs and ate them. At first, she silently denied it and shook her head in shame in an attempt not to disclose her secret. But together with the social worker we learned that for several months she had been swallowing hairs and biting her nails and swallowing them too. When I looked closely at her scalp, I saw areas of small bald spots that I had not noticed before.

"So, what do we do?" Shiri's mother asked with understandable concern.

"We'll schedule Shiri for surgery. In principle, we need to open the stomach in order to remove the hairs, they can't be removed with a gastroscopy," I explained and they sat silently opposite me in shock from the events that had progressed at a dizzying pace. To this day I remember Shiri's surgery—opening the abdomen with a small upper midline incision, grasping the enlarged stomach, making an incision along the stomach and pulling out a huge clump of hair, literally a hairball, which had blocked the entire stomach and prevented Shiri from being able to eat.

Back at the ward I catch my breath and sit for a while at the nurses' station with the shift leader, Irena, who prepares us both a cup of coffee. Relative to the mess in the ER, the ward is calm, a quiet island in the midst of immense chaos. I rest a little and let my thoughts relax. At the end of the corridor, I catch sight of Shani, the post-lumpectomy patient, walking around with an IV drip. I walk over to talk to her; it takes her a few seconds to remember who I am. Despite the late hour, her husband is here, and I explain to them what they can expect next—trying to be cautious yet optimistic—and promise that her discharge letter will be ready early in the morning. In the same room with her is Noga with the breast abscess that I drained in the ER. She has a bit of pain but overall seems fine. Irena, the nurse, calls me over.

"Mr Sa'adi from the internal ward is on his way here," she says, and I and ask her for equipment to insert a central line, recalling that two years ago Irena was with me for my first line insertion. She obviously reads my thoughts because she says, "This time it won't be like that guy with cirrhosis..."

One Friday afternoon at the start of my residency the ward was in complete chaos and I couldn't even think of going home. In the first years of general surgery residency there's no such thing as prioritizing one's private life or asking to leave early to take care of personal issues unrelated to work. Residents are expected to breathe and live the ward, burying themselves in rounds, discharge letters and admissions. On this particular Friday we were on the big round with the boss, who informed us of a new patient on the ward named Abu Moh, a 60-year-old man, seriously ill with cirrhosis, abdominal ascites and an incarcerated umbilical hernia. In principle, it's best not to operate on such patients, but in Abu Moh's case there was no escape from urgent surgery to repair the umbilical hernia, and we knew that the prognosis was not at all good. He lay panting in room 7 with a swollen abdomen. We got ready to present him to the ICU and in the meantime prepared to put him on a central line because he had almost no veins. As I was the most inexperienced resident on the ward at the time, Puta turned to me and said, "I want you to insert Abu Moh's femoral line, it's time for you to learn."

I had been thinking about the food that Gadi had prepared for me and the girls. He had just sent me a picture on WhatsApp: potatoes and sweet potatoes in the oven, and just by looking at the picture I could smell them baking. The last thing I had eaten was a dry bun from the staff room, but I had no time to dwell on food; I needed to insert a central line, one of the first skills I had to acquire during residency. Abu Moh was not a classic patient; he had coagulation disorders due to the cirrhosis and he looked in general bad condition. Puta sensed my apprehension.

"I'll be with you, Dreznik, don't worry," he reassured me. Prepare all the equipment and call me." Irena and I gathered the paraphernalia: sterile gloves, a face mask, a haircap, a kit for inserting a central line—with a triple-lumen catheter connected to one tube which is inserted into the groin—a local anesthetic, a gauze and a cleansing kit. I entered Abu Moh's room. He was a bit confused but understood when I explained to him that I would be giving him a local anesthetic on the inside of the thigh and would then insert a line into the central femoral vein, through which he would be able to receive antibiotics and fluids and other medications. I also briefly explained to him that as with any invasive operation, there is a risk of complications such as hemorrhaging or infections. Abu Moh nodded his consent to the procedure.

I suddenly had a flashback to a cadaver I examined at the National Center of Forensic Medicine who had been a homeless drug addict and had died on the street of massive blood loss when he accidently punctured the femoral artery while trying to inject drugs into the femoral vein.

I scrubbed my hands, donned a sterile gown, a hat and gloves. Puta entered the room and Irena handed me the equipment. I palpated Abu Moh's groin and felt the pulsating artery, next to where the vein should be. I anesthetized Abu Moh's thigh with lidocaine and Irena opened the kit for me that contained a huge needle, a syringe and a metal wire that I needed to thread into the vein. I made sure that the local anesthesia was working and I pricked the area where I thought the vein was, but not one drop of blood came out. I tried again, changing the angle, and a quick stream of bright blood entered the syringe, but I was a little unsure if I was in the right place.

"You've hit an artery, Dreznik," Puta said quietly, "go back in." I silently cursed myself, and as I took out the needle a few drops of arterial blood splashed in front of me. For a minute I pressed hard on the thigh and took a breather. I tried again, in a slightly different location, but still couldn't navigate to the vein, so I tried a third time, feeling a drop of blood, but it didn't flow into the syringe as it should. Next to me I heard Puta scrub his hands and don a gown, and I had a terrible feeling of failure. Puta took the syringe and needle from me, aimed a little higher and at a slightly different angle, and a stream of venous blood flowed into the syringe barrel.

Puta stopped there and let me continue the procedure which meant inserting the wire, followed by the expander, then inserting the line itself and sewing it to the skin and fixing it. I glanced several times at Abu Moh but his eyes remained closed and he lay still.

"Dreznik, you'll have plenty more opportunities, I also didn't succeed at first," Puta said, in an attempt to encourage and comfort me; he too was well familiar with the feeling of defeat.

By now I have successfully inserted dozens of central lines, including to the neck and chest, yet no matter how much experience I gain, there is always an element of self-doubt coupled with the memory of my mini-failures, including Abu Moh. But I no longer dwell on this, I have reconciled with my past and now look ahead to even greater challenges that await me.

10 p.m.

"Listen, I need a favor from you," I say on the phone to our on-call gastroenterologist, Maor, after looking at the abdominal x-ray of my friend Alon Zinger, who Shpet has nicknamed 'Alon love egg' after I told him of my bizarre encounter with him in the ER. Maor answers from home and I hear him yelling at his kids to go to sleep.

"I have a young man here with an egg stuck in his rectum, about halfway up. It can't be removed and I need your help." I hear Maor's thoughts—*it's not urgent and can wait till morning*—but I try my luck anyway.

"It doesn't sound urgent," Maor says, unsurprisingly. "Get him hospitalized and we'll do a colonoscopy in the morning." I know that Alon will never agree to be hospitalized; the fear of his wife finding out outweighs the reasonable option for him to stay the night with us.

"Can I schedule him an urgent examination for the morning and discharge him in the meantime, in terms of hospital obligation and so forth?" I ask, trying my luck a second time. Maor answers in the affirmative, as though aware that this is a delicate situation that required discretion. I schedule an examination for the following morning, then return to the ER to update Alon. He and the woman next to him are exchanging tense glances. They probably had an argument about the whole incident, but right now I have no time to preoccupy myself with the juicy details. I instruct Alon to fast and write him a temporary discharge letter. Irena texts me that Mr Sa'adi is on his way to room 2 on the ward and that the blood units have arrived and are heated, ready to be connected to the central line. She also informs me that Kamal, the nurse in charge of room 2, will be with me during the procedure.

I really like Kamal. We have been good friend since the start of my residency. In fact, we started our rotation in general surgery together—he in nursing and I in medicine. His dream is to become a doctor and is he hoping to pass his third psychometric test. He is young and intelligent with a lot of determination and patience and I have no doubt that one day he will get accepted to medical school, even though the road is long and sometimes discouraging. Kamal and I meet in the staff room on the ward, just before the hospital orderly moves Mr Sa'adi to his bed and the nurses take vital signs. I ask Kamal about his psychometric.

"I'm studying so hard and I'm fed up, but I have no choice," he replies, and I try to give him words of encouragement.

I remember the sheer joy I felt when I was accepted to medical school. Many children dream of being a doctor when they grow up and every nursery school is equipped with a toy medical kit so that children can play at pretending to be doctors and nurses. As adults, anatomy and physiology hold a fascination for many of us and we all understand the benefits of first aid and CPR training so that we can respond in a medical emergency and help save lives. But I never imagined I would be a doctor; it was the furthest thing from my mind... that is, until I was 26 years old.

I think it all started one day when I was on my way to Jerusalem to my former job as an economist at the Ministry of Finance. It was a long journey and I had a lot of time to think while admiring the stunning Jerusalem Hills in front of me. And then it just hit me. Like Neo, the protagonist of *The Matrix*, whose reality becomes foggy and he realizes that he's living in a kind of dream, I too tried to see through the fog and realized that this was not the reality I wanted to live for the rest of my life. But I couldn't explain to myself why medicine was calling out to me. The desire to become a doctor landed on me without warning or explanation, like a five-ton stone churning in my stomach. And once the realization hit with full force, there was no turning back.

Tamar was six months old at the time. I remember buying a psychometric test kit with trembling hands and registering for the test. I thought my chances of doing well in the test were slim; in high school I neglected my studies and my grades were way below the minimum threshold for acceptance to university. But I was very motivated and determined, so I ploughed my way through one psychometric test after another and retook high school courses in order to improve my grades, spending entire weekends learning verses of the Bible, historical facts and math equations. This went on for two long years, at the end of which all my hard work paid off when I finally got accepted to medical school. I honestly don't know what I would have done had I not been accepted. Kamal likes to hear this story again and again; it gives him hope and incentive to persevere, despite the fact that the entry criteria for medical school have become more stringent.

Kamal and I finish talking, and I receive a text message from Alon, who is saved in my contacts as 'Alon Egg'.

You're the best! he texts. *I'm coming tomorrow morning for a colonoscopy. I will never forget what you've done for me.* I smile, put my phone back in my pocket and go to meet Mr Sa'adi.

Mr Sa'adi is in his 60s and on dialysis as a result of kidney disease from a young age, which in recent years has developed and worsened. He also suffers from hemorrhoids, and the combination of blood thinners, dialysis and hemorrhoids is probably what caused the significant bleeding. Earlier, while he was on the internal ward, the internists called the surgeons for a consultation, so by the time Johnny got to him, Mr Sa'adi had already bled a considerable amount, and his blood pressure, which was already quite low, had dropped even more. His heart rate was up and he looked paler than usual.

The first thing I notice about him is his wonderful open smile that connotes good nature and kindness. Like Aharon on the ward, Mr Sa'adi and I instantly connect and form a special and rare bond. He is concerned about his wife, who came to the hospital as soon as she heard he was bleeding and has been running to hospitals with him for years, taking care of him, always by his side for better, for worse, for richer, for poorer, in sickness and in health.

Kamal and I prepare the equipment and I connect two doses of blood to the line. I execute everything in the exact same way I tried to execute it with Abu Moh, only this time I do it swiftly and skillfully, like riding a bicycle. I puncture the vein, go straight in with the applicator, insert the line, then suture the line to the inner skin of the thigh.

Kamal and I check that Sa'adi's details match those of the blood infusion and start giving Sa'adi the first dose. It's almost 11 p.m. and ward is quiet. All the visitors have left, but Mr Sa'adi's wife stays for a while, wanting to make sure that everything is okay. He has stopped bleeding from his rectum for now—the Gelfoam is helping—but if the bleeding returns, he'll need urgent surgery.

I finish dressing Mr Sa'adi's line area and then remember that while rushing around I forgot to call home and say goodnight to the girls. They are probably asleep by now, Gadi too. Too often during shifts I have a fleeting pang of guilt when I realize that my opportunity to call home has slipped by. Other times, Gadi will call me and I talk quickly and briefly because I have no time to chat. I compensate myself by planning how I will spend tomorrow afternoon with the girls. Perhaps I'll make them lunch or order in, as I've been doing too often lately. Then we'll watch a movie together and I'll smother them with hugs and kisses.

I take out my phone again and slide the screen with my fingers that are still coated in a thin layer of talc from the sterile gloves. There's a WhatsApp message from Gadi, with a short rundown on today's events: *Hi, Yael, Nitzan and I sat through Tamar's ballet class, then we bought cookies and snacks. They danced in the living room and were good girls. Hope all is quiet there, have a good shift.* I smile, yet feel a twinge of sadness that I didn't talk to my girls before bed. I debate whether to text Gadi back since it's late, but decide to write a few words. He always laughs at my laconic replies when I'm at work, such as: *It's hard* or *I'm tired*, so I try to elaborate a little more now.

Thinking about lunch tomorrow with the girls is a reminder that I haven't eaten a proper meal today, and as if Shpet had read my thoughts, he suddenly calls me and invites me to the residents' room for pizza. I feel my stomach juices churning as I head to the residents' room, the smell of hot pizza drifting into the ward. I see Johnny take two triangles of pizza and fold them into a cone, and hear Shpet mumble something with his mouth full. We eat ravenously, urgently gorging on the pizza, our fuel, while we again discuss the ER. Shpet is concerned about a 90-year-old man, named Weitzner, who came to the ER with abdominal pain and an intestinal obstruction due to a tumor that has just been discovered in an abdominal CT scan. As we eat, Shpet calls our on-call attending.

"Hi, Dr Cohen," says Shpet, "sorry to disturb you, but we have a 90-year-old man in the ER with high blood pressure and diabetes, he's fully conscious and completely lucid. In short, he's had abdominal pain for a few days now, says he's a little constipated. His last colonoscopy was over 10 years ago. The enema CT we just did shows an obstructing tumor in the left colon, we can't see metastases and the small intestine is not dilated." Johnny and I glance at each other; we know where this is going—a complete colon obstruction means immediate surgery.

11 p.m.

I remember our family trip to Abel Tasman National Park on the south coast of New Zealand, just before my internship started. Nitzan was only four then, Tamar eight, and the deep blue ocean stretched out in front of us. We were on a small motorboat that made foam and waves. Nitzan sat on my lap with a life jacket, she and Tamar giggling every time the boat jumped a little. The sun's bright golden rays shone on the three of us and I held this moment frozen in the air, a moment so happy that it physically hurt, and I didn't want it to end. I had just finished my studies, we were on the other side of the world, and at night in our caravan I reflected on all the things I needed to do before my internship, such as open a file at the Ministry of Health and go to the hospital for an orientation day.

Every so often the memories of Abel Tasman come to mind, and I don't know why I am thinking of them now, as Mr Weitzner with the colon obstruction finishes a dose of intravenous morphine. Perhaps because of the unfathomable fragility of life.

Our attending, Dr Cohen, arrives at the hospital to talk to Mr Weitzner, who has just been transferred to the ward. Mr Weitzner has the tanned, wrinkled skin of someone who has spent many years in the sun; pigmentation and old age spots cover his hands and face. His son and daughter arrive and look at their father bleary-eyed, not sure how this mess came about. Weitzner was born in Poland and immigrated to Israel before WW2. For years he has been living in an assisted living facility with a caregiver, and he is still lucid but only partially independent. More and more people aged 90 and older are now coming to us for surgery with an inguinal hernia, cholecystitis[8] or intestinal tumors. Some time ago I prepared a statistical analysis for the boss on the average age of cholecystitis among patients on the ward and we discovered that most of them are over the age of 75, and the older the patient, the greater the risk that the

---

[8] Inflammation of the gallbladder.

disease will lead to life-threatening complications. In some cases, we assist seriously ill patients in ending their life, and although this is not within the scope of a doctor's role, it often seems to me like the right thing to do.

"I don't want surgery," Mr Weitzner says firmly. The morphine is still working and he is in less pain for now. Cohen and Shpet again explain the situation to Mr Weitzner and his children. Shpet speaks gently and softly.

"You have an obstructing tumor in your colon," he says, "and without surgery, the pressure created in the digestive system will eventually cause a hole in the colon and lead to a fatal abdominal infection."

The son and daughter are very confused. They don't know the statistics and what the chances are of their 90-year-old father recovering from surgery; what the quality of his life will be, assuming that the surgery goes smoothly. I myself am not even sure of the odds. The latest medical literature with regard to surgery among nonagenarians is fairly optimistic and indicates they have a high chance of recovery, a high life expectancy and a good postoperative quality of life.

"Mr Weitzner," says Cohen, "I can't decide for you, we will of course respect your decision. It's important that you know that we are available for you at any hour should you decide on surgery."

I look at Mr Weitzner. He doesn't look at us, just caresses the edge of the sheet that wraps him, and an oppressive silence prevails. My mind once again escapes, uninvited, to the sunshine of Abel Tasman.

After the conversation with Mr Weitzner, Shpet, Johnny and I sit in the residents' room for a few minutes and Shpet documents the conversation on the computer.
"We have to operate on him," Shpet suddenly says with strong conviction, and I know where this sentiment is coming from: A 95-year-old patient named Shimonov, who was recently the subject of a heated debate in the department.

The story of Shiminov began three months ago. He had lung disease, was confined to a wheelchair and had 24/7 nursing care. He was lucid, despite moments of confusion and he had been coming to the internal ward every month to receive blood and iron transfusions for anemia. Due to his age, he did not undergo a colonoscopy, but when he began to lose a significant amount of blood and his hemoglobin level dropped to 6 g/dL, a comprehensive investigation was carried out and a huge tumor was found in his transverse colon that was causing the bleeding. A meeting was held to discuss how to proceed with the case, attended by the director of the department, all the senior doctors and Shpet. *What should we do? Should we operate? What surgery? Should we do a stoma?* A minority of the doctors were opposed to operating on Shiminov, and it was agreed to do only minimal surgery: tumor resection and transverse colostomy, in the hope that in his current condition he would come out of it safely. We explained the situation to Shimonov's family and it was hard for them to make a decision, but in the end agreed to the surgery. For my part, I didn't know what was best to do.

I was chosen to assist in the surgery, and I remember laying Shimonov on the operating table with extreme care, like a newborn baby. He was so frail, bled from every IV insertion and had hematomas in every part of his body. The surgery was a miraculous success with minimal complications, and two weeks later Shimonov was discharged home. After his last visit to the clinic, he no longer needed blood transfusions. So as Shpet documents the conversation with Mr Weitzner, he feels confident that surgery will save Weitzner's life too.

I have some respite from the ER, where there's a woman with suspected appendicitis waiting for an abdominal CT and two other elderly patients who had a head CT due to a fall, and I'm waiting for the results in the hope that I can send them home. Johnny is with a patient in the trauma unit and Shpet informs the OR that Mr Weitzner may have urgent surgery tonight. I go out into the ward corridor and see Dana, Aviad's wife bringing him a cup of tea. She immediately recognizes me and we smile at each other. We talk about her middle son's upcoming Bar Mitzvah and their recent vacation overseas with the whole family. Dana tells me that she and Aviad met during their army service and have been together ever since.

"I chased after him and eventually won him over," she says with a twinkle in her eye. She invites me for a cigarette and a coffee tomorrow morning, then I go into Aviad's room with her. It has three beds, Aviad's facing the window. The other two patients are asleep and Aviad looks so out of place here. "Take it, SpongeBob," Dana says with a chuckle, as she hands her husband the tea, then leaves to get something from the nurses' station. Aviad is sitting cross-legged on the bed with one arm hanging loosely on a knee. He looks at me inquisitively and I wait for his question.

"Tell me, Dr Yael," he says, "if we assume that my jaundice is not due to gallstones, then what could it be?"

"I hesitate. "It...it could be a tumor," I finally reply. How I hate having to say those words. But I can't lie to him, even though the chances of him having a tumor are slim since he's only 45 years old. The words float in the air. Aviad lifts his arm off his knee and slowly drops his head to his chest, and I am grateful that Dana had not yet returned.

I take a deep breath of the night air and shiver a little in the October chill, thinking about my conversation with Aviad and the look in his eyes. I hope he'll be okay. I try to put it out of my mind as I make my way to the ER again to discharge a few patients, check on a young soldier complaining of heartburn, suture the wound of a man who fell and cut his forehead, and examine a returning Crohn's patient who now has abdominal pain. Meanwhile, Mr Weitzner begins to complain of pain again; it's been half an hour since his intravenous morphine was stopped. The nurses call Shpet and he returns to the ward to once again talk to the family. Mr Weitzner's resolve not to go to the OR begins to wane as his abdominal pain worsens and in the end he and family agree to surgery.

"Weitzner 's in pain, we're going to the OR," Johnny informs me. "Try to finish things up in the ER and come watch. In the meantime, I'm going to scrub in with Shpet and Cohen," he says. I know this means that I will now be alone again in the trauma unit and the ER, but this is how it is.

Midnight

Mr Weitzner's children say goodbye to him at the entrance to the OR, tilting their heads in deep concern. As I briskly walk to the ER to check what else is left to finish up, I see Shpet, Johnny and Cohen go into the OR. As I sit down in my chair in room 4 for the hundredth time, I feel fatigue seep into every muscle of my body. It's a minute after midnight, the date on the clock has changed, and by this point I am counting down the hours till I go home. I finish discharging two patients with minor head injuries, and things quieten down a little. The ER itself is crowded; this is the time when people arrive: casualties of car accidents with limb injuries, the elderly from nursing homes and people with chest pains, and the triage area is now fully-staffed.

I have patients waiting in the triage area for blood tests and more imaging, but they are all closed in terms of initial management, so I make myself a coffee and drink it quickly, tempted to believe that the caffeine will boost my energy for the next few hours. On my phone I open Skandalakis' Surgical Anatomy app—our surgical guidebook—which details with great accuracy the stages in common general surgeries, and I read a little about the colectomy, or colon resection surgery, that Mr Weitzner is about to undergo.

One day, long before I dreamt of becoming a doctor, I found myself at Tel Aviv university's Faculty of Medicine walking along a path surrounded by green lawns, the sun beating down on my head, even though it was January when it's usually cold. My first semester exams in economics were about to begin, yet there I was, at the Faculty of Medicine, not knowing why my legs had carried me there, not realizing it was a prelude of things to come. On the board at the entrance to the faculty was a chart of all the study material for the anatomy exam, which I skimmed in disbelief, then swiftly made my way back along the path and out of the campus. I returned a few years later, after a period of upheaval in my life, determined to come to terms with medicine, the mountain of material to learn and the hundreds of names of muscles, tendons, organs and vasculature that I needed to memorize for the anatomy exam at the end of the first semester. I read, analyzed and summarized the material, made tables, summarized again, made up acronyms, then forgot them. I wasn't alone in the uphill battle against an onslaught of information—all the students were drowning in infinity, their brain overloaded with details, painfully starved of oxygen.

I have a picture in my mind of me and Zehavit on our first day of medical school sitting with a box of bones we received in anatomy class—a skull, a humerus and spine bones—trying to remember the Latin names for their different parts, closing our eyes and testing each other over and over, an almost Sisyphean task. In addition to the harrowing anatomy exam, there was the pharmacology exam in third year with a million medications to remember, including side effects and drug interactions. Two weeks later was the bacteriology exam for which we had to memorize all the bacteria, viruses, fungi and parasites that exist, their mechanisms of attack and resistance. The entire second year was dedicated to the study of the various body systems, starting with the cardiovascular system and ending with the most difficult—for me at least—the urinary system. And by then I was in my ninth month with Nitzan. My brain was empty and swollen, yet I pass the exam by the skin of my teeth. And when our studies finished there were the final exams; six grueling months of insurmountable pressure, endless summaries, books and questions, until I started to experience burnout and felt that I was running on an empty tank.

This endless learning continues throughout my professional life and never stops. And so it is with us all: Johnny who passed the first stage exams in general surgery last June after reading almost a thousand pages of a book on general surgery and answering questions that dealt with the tiniest details; Shpet who is now studying for his final oral exams—stage two; our senior doctors who write research papers and read the latest articles in their field; and I, here in the ER reading Skandalakis' Surgical Anatomy, trying to understand what complications can arise in left colon resection surgery. And I suddenly think fondly of Mrs Segal whom I met a year ago, wondering how she is doing and greatly missing her.

Mrs Segal was a tough, opinionated and domineering 80-year-old woman with sharp eyes, an aquiline nose and a mischievous smile. She came to the ER complaining of changes in her bowel habits. We admitted her to the ward and found a tumor in her right colon, which required a colectomy—bowel resection surgery. After months and months of performing minor ambulatory surgeries such as breast biopsies and inguinal hernias, bowel resection is considered a resident's first major surgery, so I obviously felt very privileged when I learned that I was going to perform the surgery with the boss as the attending surgeon.

The night before, I brushed up on my anatomy and memorized the blood supply, trying to imagine what questions the boss might ask me during the surgery. But more than anything I was very excited.

"She is not an easy woman, Dreznik," the boss told me, with a knowing smile. I had heard about Mrs Segal also from Puta who admitted her at the preoperative clinic.

"She's no fool, a tough lady," Puta warned me, leaving me to face her alone in the preoperative waiting room. But to my surprise, Mrs Segal and I immediately established a good rapport. I may have reminded her of her granddaughter who she told me had gone overseas. Just before we entered the OR she grabbed my hand very tightly, looked at me with her sharp eyes and said in a commanding voice: "Look after me in the OR, I'm no spring chicken." I smiled at her and didn't let go of her hand until the anesthesiologist had put her to sleep.

The boss let me do the whole surgery skin-to-skin. We cut out the large tumor located in the area of the hepatic flexure, checked there were no metastases in the abdomen and anastomosed the remaining intestine. I worked slowly—this was after all my first major surgery—and tied all the threads well to make sure there was no bleeding or leakage. I wanted zero complications, even though I was aware that her age and her large tumor didn't play in her favor. I had promised her I would look after her.

The day after the surgery I had the day off, but decided to drop by the ward to visit Mrs Segal and check that she was urinating and feeling good. She began to slowly recover and was able to eat a little and move around the ward with a walker and the help of the physiotherapist. But then on the fifth day, as though she had read Skandalakis' book, she developed a slight fever and her abdominal pain worsened. In medical jargon this is called suspected anastomotic leakage, whereby the connection made during surgery between the parts of the bowel loosen and feces spill into the abdominal cavity, causing an intra-abdominal infection. This occurred just at the end of a shift when I was worn out and wanted to go home, but Mrs Segal's sharp, suffering eyes gave me no rest.

"Dr Yael, I don't feel so well today," she said to me. I quickly arranged for an abdominal CT scan and the result confirmed my biggest concern—a leak in the area of the anastomosis; not big, but a leak nevertheless. I informed the boss and he too was very upset and disappointed, but there was nothing we could do. We started Mrs Segal on intravenous antibiotics, told her to fast and hoped for the best. When I eventually got home, I knew that if her condition worsened, I would have to return to the hospital, no matter how tired I was, and reoperate on her. The hours passed slowly, I was anxious and unable to sleep until late at night when I received a call from the on-call doctor on the ward who notified me that Mrs Segal was doing well.

The days passed and Mrs Segal slowly recovered during two long weeks of hospitalization. The day she was discharged, she kissed me on both cheeks and said, "Dr Yael, come and visit me at home and we'll play the piano together."

I quietly enter the OR, just as Cohen, Johnny and Shpet are deep inside Mr Weitzner's abdomen. The nurses glance over at me, the anesthesiologist is engrossed in vitals, and there is silence, broken only by the buzz of the diathermy, the beeping of the monitor and the rustle of blood-stained gloves deep inside the intestines. I sit on a stool and peep inside, being careful not to undo the sterility.

"Continue along this area, the tumor is here, stuck to the spleen," Cohen tells Shpet. They become aware of my presence and begin to explain a little: "A small tumor, but it has caused a full obstruction," Johnny tells me through his mask. I see them holding the left colon, which is starting to separate from its blood supply, and I see the area with the stubborn tumor, part of which is breaking out, stuck to the spleen. I remember what I read earlier in Skandalakis' chapter on left colon resection, how this part is one of the most problematic due to its proximity to the spleen. And just as Mrs Segal had seemingly read in Skandalakis' book that an anastomotic leak presents on the fifth day after surgery, so it now seems as if Mr Weitzner has read Skandalakis' chapter about splenic bleeding during left colon separation. I hear Cohen mutter, "Shit," and realize that Mr Weitzner is in trouble.

1 a.m.

"This is the most bipolar profession there is, Dreznik. Some day you'll understand what I mean," Shpet said, sharing with me yet another of his insights that stay with me to this day. That was at the start of my residency, and now I understand what he meant, as he holds Mr Weitzner 's colon and the capsule of the spleen that is still bleeding despite attempts to stop it. I hear Cohen telling the nurses and the anesthesiologist that they should prepare for a splenectomy.

I first heard the term bipolar disorder during my psychiatry rotation as a student. It well described Rachel, the first patient I interviewed in the psychiatric daycare hospital.

I began my psychiatric rotation in my fifth year of medical school. The psychiatric building is far from the main hospital, as though cut off from it. Surrounding it are green lawns and inside there is a huge lobby. It was still cold outside at 8 a.m. on my first day and an overcast sky hinted of rain as I entered the building with great trepidation and curiosity. I had already done rotations in internal medicine, general surgery, pediatrics and gynecology and learned how to identify heart murmurs, scrub in for surgery, perform a full physical examination on premature babies, deliver a baby both naturally and by caesarean section, perform a rectal examination and take blood samples. But there is nothing quite like the experience of psychiatry rotation; all other departments are alike, but the psychiatric department is different in its own way.

Miri, a good friend from medical school who was doing this rotation with me, was waiting for me on one of the comfortable armchairs in the lobby. We drank coffee, talked a little about our studies and agreed that our psychiatry rotation hours where better than our gynecology rotation hours which began at 7:15 a.m.
We continued to chat, when suddenly a young woman, large and clumsy, stormed into the lobby and banged her head seven times on the bathroom door. We looked away in

horror. "Welcome to the psychiatry rotation," Miri said apprehensively, and we suspected that the young woman suffered from obsessive compulsive disorder, which later turned out to be true.

The first session with a psychiatric patient is called an 'intake' at which the psychiatrist gathers basic information about the patient, and it can last an hour or two. At our first intake, Miri and I and the psychiatrist sat opposite a young patient in his 2os named Roy. He told us that he had a normal childhood but began having difficulties in the army. He had discipline issues, liked to be alone, believed that he was special and had an important role in the world. He spent time in a military prison for disobeying orders and after his release he couldn't find himself. He told us that at the age of 21 an inner voice told him that he was destined to redeem people, a little like the biblical heroes but in a completely different constellation. Roy talked about his first psychotic episode during which he had visions and heard voices talking to him. Everything in his stories seemed so real that I still remember them years later.

Miri and I were fascinated, mesmerized, and as the intake session progressed and we got deeper inside Roy's turbulent mind, he told us that during one of his psychotic episodes he almost killed someone because he heard voices telling him that this was the only way to redemption.

By lunch time my mouth was dry from listening to Roy, the first schizophrenic patient I met. I went to the staff kitchen, drank some cold water and let my thoughts rest. I imagined how I would tell Gadi about all these stories, why psychiatry is so interesting, and that maybe I should abandon surgery in favor of mental illness.

By the end of my first week of psychiatry rotation my brain was bursting with information about schizophrenia, depression, anxiety disorders, personality disorders and an endless list of medications. Miri and I would visit the closed psychiatric ward at a later stage. In the meantime, we got to know the patients who came for day treatment, the balanced patients who led a relatively independent life but needed the medical support provided by the department.

One day I was asked to interview Rachel, a well-groomed woman in her sixties, who wore a tailored jacket and a delicate, colorful scarf around her neck. I could easily imagine her as my mother. She told me about her life—her office job, children, husband, financial worries, and her spells of mild depression, which all sounded normal. But then she told me about her first manic episode at the age of 40. She would go on shopping sprees and walk for hours on end as though someone was chasing her. She would sleep three hours a night and wake up refreshed, as if she was on stimulants. Her husband didn't understand what had happened to her, where all the money had gone, and why there was an endless pile of shopping bags. Her family thought that she might have a shopping addiction, but then she suddenly fell into depression. Most of the day she slept, didn't get up for work, had a low mood and spent most of her time alone. A few years later she had another manic episode that involved petty gambling. This went on for many years until she was eventually diagnosed with bipolar disorder and was treated with medication and psychiatric day care. I talked to her about the disorder and asked her how she was coping. I had a sense that something in her was lost. She smiled at times, was serious at times, but mainly there was an emptiness in her facial expressions which was hard for me to put my finger on. She tried to convey to me what it feels like to be in mania, when the whole world is dancing around you, and then later everything comes crashing down, and I had a feeling that she was missing these emotional ups and downs, because that day she was in a kind of fog, like a straight line, void of ups and downs.

Surgeons can also experience this sharp transition from mania to depression, often in one day, a few hours apart, and there is no cure for it. For instance, a week ago, a child came to the ER with appendicitis. I operated on him towards the end of my shift and it was a difficult procedure with lots of adhesions and an abscess around the appendix. Yet I managed to remove the appendix laparoscopically and the attending surgeon congratulated me on a job well done. The child's parents were thrilled and I naturally felt on top of the world. But the following morning, at a meeting with all the senior doctors, the boss reprimanded me for forgetting to schedule another patient an important preoperative examination. In that moment I felt breathless, small, humiliated, and my euphoria since the appendectomy the day before suddenly washed away in a flood of disappointment. These extremes of exhilaration one minute and devastation the next, are hard to fathom.

I see Shpet's eyes peeping over his surgical mask. He disconnects Weitzner's bleeding spleen from its attachments, and with a stapler he closes the splenic blood vessels and ligates the splenic artery and vein. His forehead is beaded with sweat. Two days ago, Shpet saved the life of a patient with a bowel obstruction, and now Weitzner is under his knife, hanging between life and death. Just a couple of hours ago Shpet held Weitzner 's hand and told him that there was no escape from surgery to save his life, and now this truth is crumbling before our eyes. I know that Shpet is feeling the bipolarity, the constant swinging back and forth like a pendulum between joy and fear.

I stay in the OR a while longer. There is an update from the ER that another elderly woman who fell today has arrived with abdominal pain and hematoma. But I am waiting to see what happens with Weitzner, his abdomen wide open, spread out in front of us on this night of intestinal loops, a bleeding spleen and the smell of diathermy. I'm beginning to realize that Weitzner's chances of escaping this peril are slim, but I can't quite digest it. Shpet, Cohen and Johnny work quickly and quietly in an atmosphere of desperation. They finish separating the tumor, the bleeding has stopped and the tumor is out. But the anesthesiologist is not satisfied with Weitzner's urine output and the result of his blood gas test. There are now signs of acidosis in the blood; Weitzner's body is betraying him. At the age of 90 he obviously knew why he didn't want surgery.

I leave the OR, trying to avoid Weitzner's anxious children in the waiting room. Back in the ER I answer a call from a pediatrician in the pediatric ER.

"Hi, is this the on-call surgeon?" he asks. "I have a month-old baby here with an incarcerated inguinal hernia. He's vomiting."

2 a.m.

I head to the pediatric unit, watching the moon shimmer on the hospital buildings. How many times have I been in this darkness with my thoughts, waiting for morning to come, afraid of what the night still holds? This moment reminds me of a song by Soulsavers called "Longest Day". I first heard the song at the start of my internship while sipping coffee one night during my third shift in the internal medicine department. The ward was full of ventilated patients in critical condition, filling me with a sense of impending doom. Ofir, a resident, played the song on his phone and sang along to it while he wrote admission notes. Since then the words have stuck in my head:

I was walking home alone

Late the other night

I couldn't see a single star in the sky

Oh, they must be too high

Shadows dance around me in the dark

Don't stop

This could be the longest day

And the night has yet to come

It's hot outside, even though it's the middle of the night, but I'm a little cold from lack of sleep. I pray there won't be any more major surprises tonight. All the patients I have seen today, examined, treated and operated on are shadows in the darkness, dancing around me in slow motion, and all I want to do is lie down and close my eyes. There are three well-known "rules" that are instilled into the psyche of surgical residents: "Sleep when you can, eat when you can, and don't mess with the pancreas." Before they did renovations on the ER, there were four rooms for the night shifts, which were always somehow occupied, so I would wander around the intermediate care units, dragging my tired legs, in search of an empty bed. Or I would sleep on a children's bed at the entrance to the pediatric OR, squashed in a supine position. Sometimes there were no sheets or pillows so I'd put my hoodie under my head, praying that the pager wouldn't ring with its shrill cry and end my nap. Once, I didn't get a chance to sleep until 5:45 a.m., a quarter of an hour before the morning round. I sat on a chair near the enema room in the back entrance of the ER, laid my head back and was out like a light.

I arrive at the pediatric ER and hear a lot of commotion in one of the rooms next to the triage.

"The surgeon has arrived," I hear the pediatrician inform the baby's parents, who throw me a look that expresses a whole range of emotions: fear, concern, the feeling that everything depends on me now; I am the savior on whom their son's life depends.

A little baby boy about a month old is lying on the bed. Every time I examine small babies it reminds me of where I want to be down the road: in pediatric surgery. How I adore the pink, soft body of a baby that has yet to learn so much of life. How I love a baby's innocent smile that never fails to brighten up my day. I'm always amazed how quickly infants recover from cancer, difficult surgeries, congenital anomalies, and how everything about them is authentic. And when they love, it's the purest love there is.

The baby's parents look young and I'm sure it's their first child. There is something vulnerable about being a first-time parent and this vulnerability fills the air in the room, you can't miss it. Despite my fatigue, I summon up all the empathy I can muster to deal with the task at hand. While I undress the baby and take off his diaper, I ask the parents when he was born, if he was premature and if there is anything of importance regarding his medical background. I don't have time to look at them or to make polite conversation; the hernia needs to be reduced, and quickly. In a potentially urgent case such as this, I don't delay too much in taking the anamnesis, but go straight to a physical examination. I immediately identify an incarcerated inguinal hernia on the right side of the groin where there is an unmistakable bulge. In my two years of residency, I have seen many incarcerated hernias among infants and the very elderly. This is one of the first skills a general surgeon must learn, because if the hernia cannot be manually maneuvered back inside the abdomen, emergency surgery is necessary. So the surgeon's goal will always be to buy time before elective hernia repair surgery later on, which is often preferable to emergency surgery in terms of its results and potential complications.

About six months into my residency, the internist in ER called me and asked me to examine an elderly man with an incarcerated hernia. At the ER, I saw a huge bulge in the patient's groin which I tried, without success, to maneuver back into the abdomen. I remember the man moaning in pain, so I gave him some morphine and tried again, but to no avail. In the end I called Imrish, who with his "magic" maneuver and some strength managed to do a successful manual reduction and push the hernia sac back into place. For me, this was similar to my experience with Abu Moh and the femoral line; an overwhelming feeling of failure accompanied by fierce determination to do better next time.

I hold the bulge in the little baby's groin and feel the testicle below it, making sure it's not undescended. I feel the external ring of the inguinal canal and maneuver the hernia back into the abdomen until the bulge disappears and the baby calms down. The procedure literally takes seconds, like a magic trick. The parents look on in wonder, the pediatrician smiles and I quietly celebrate my small victory, collecting another small medal on this shift. I explain to the parents what a hernia is, why elective surgery is needed and what to expect next. They can't thank me enough.

I don't always remember the medals I collect during shifts, because the things that go wrong tend to overshadow the things that go right. However, even when my successes don't seem that important at the time, I try to stop for a moment at the end of each shift and reflect on them. This shift, for instance, began with a surgery to remove Shani's breast tumor; then my meeting with Smadar in the ambulatory clinic where she gave me chocolates; a good lecture with the medical students;

intussusception reduction on baby Yuval (which reminds me that I have to visit him in the morning and see how he's doing); my insistence on a CT scan for Osnat and correctly diagnosing her; my immediate connection with Aviad and his wife; drainage of Noga's breast abscess; suturing incisions, insertion of a femoral line and stabilization of Sa'adi who was bleeding; and now this successful manual reduction of an incarcerated hernia.

By the time I finish writing a consultation report in the pediatric ER, it is already 2:45 a.m. I glance at the ER dashboard to check if the elderly woman with abdominal pain and hematoma is still waiting for me, and maybe after checking on her I can finally get some sleep. Just then Shpet texts me: *We've finished the laparotomy, an awful surgery. Close the dashboard in the ER and abort.* I think of Mr Weitzner and imagine the conversation that Shpet, Cohen and Johnny must be having with his children right now: *It was a difficult surgery, he is in poor condition and the next few hours are critical.* Until a moment ago I was counting medals and filing them away deep in my heart, but now the Soulsavers' song is looping in my head and I can't see a single star in the sky.

I head back to the ER while Shpet goes to the ward to make sure that everyone is asleep, including our asterisks. When I was still an intern, he took me with him on one of these quick rounds which he likes to call 'Shpet's blitz', and since then I often do the same, especially when I am alone on the ward. Later he'll tell me about his conversation with Weitzner's family and we'll go to the recovery room to check on Weitzner, only to see him fade away along with his blood pressure, which is gradually dropping, signaling his departure from this life. Shpet walks down the long, dark corridor of the ward to check on Aaron and gently turns on the light in his room. Aharon's wife is sleeping next to him and Shpet slowly opens the curtain to look at the drains. In one of them there is a drop of blood. He looks at the monitor; Aharon's blood pressure is good and his pulse is normal. Shpet squeezes the drain and no more blood comes out. He instructs the nurses to keep an eye on Aaron, hoping the bleeding is only temporary, and goes to sleep.

3 a.m.

Mrs Konigsberg is a small, chubby lady. I meet her at the entrance to the ER, and she knows I've come to examine her because on my way to the pediatric ER to check on the baby with the incarcerated hernia, Omri, the internist in the ER, had casually introduced her to me.

"She fell tonight while getting on a bus and bruised her lower right chest and upper right abdomen," Omri says. "She fell from a standing height, nothing serious, and she's not taking blood thinners. It's just that she's complaining of pain, so I'm thinking of sending her home with some pain killers." I have known Omri since we did internship together in the pediatric department. He is a talented doctor with a lot of knowledge, mostly theoretical, but when it comes to the clinical understanding of a patient, he is a little less experienced in my opinion. We surgeons work closely with the interns and nurses in the chaos of the ER, and there are those among them who if they tell you that a patient doesn't look good, you drop everything and run. But there are others who you sometimes need to take what they say with a grain of salt. Omri falls into the latter group, so I was skeptical of his opinion. I asked him to send Mrs Konigsberg for lab tests and he pulls a familiar sullen face.

"What do you expect us to do with lab tests? he persisted. It'll only keep her stuck here for another hour and the woman's dying to go home. Besides, her son is breathing down my neck."

I understood Omri, but I explained to him that I wanted to be sure. This mild hematoma below the lower right rib may indeed not be serious, but sometimes my instincts tell me to be careful. Even though Mrs Konigsberg doesn't want to do blood tests, she in nevertheless in a lot of pain.

On my return from the pediatric ER, I go room 4, and before inviting Mrs Konigsberg in I take a look at her lab tests and find that her liver functions are very elevated which could be the result of a liver laceration when she fell or a chronic condition. But I don't have any previous tests to compare them to. I call the radiologist, knowing there's a good chance he's asleep and will curse me for waking him to request an abdominal CT. I silently mutter to myself: *If there is any doubt, there is no doubt.*

A few years back, a month after my internship, I went with all the family to Tel Aviv University for my M.D. graduation ceremony. 120 future doctors stood in a huge hall, clad in black robes and hats, and as the dean of our faculty read aloud the physician's oath, we all raised our hand in the air, solemnly swearing to uphold the oath. There was something sacred in that moment that I wanted to capture and freeze in my memory, so that I could conjure it up every time something clouded my judgment, my professionalism, my humanity.

I took Nitzan and Tamar up to the stage with me to receive my diploma and shake hands with all the heads of the Faculty of Medicine. My two little redheads bounced excitedly onto the stage, making me so proud of them. After the ceremony I walked alone to my car that was parked on the other side of the university, watching a summer cloud disperse in the sky. I got into the car, started the engine, leaned my head on the steering wheel and cried with joy. A few days earlier I had formulated a list of ten medical 'commandments' for myself which I hoped would light my way through internship, residency and my entire medical career. One of them is: *If there is a doubt, there is no doubt*, a rule I decided to always abide by after I once violated it with a patient—despite having doubts—and regret it to this day.

So, in Mrs Konigsberg's case, I suspect that she may have a liver injury, so that when Roy the radiologist answers my call, I have to convince him that she needs an abdominal CT scan.

"You're crazy, Dreznik, enough of your scans already!" the radiologist barks at me. I hear his tiredness and know exactly how he feels; we are all in the same rickety boat at 3:30 a.m. "Earlier," he continues, "Johnny asked me to do an abdominal CT for a woman he thought had appendicitis and she didn't have anything, and now at 4 a.m. you want me to do a CT scan for some little old lady with mild abdominal hematoma who fell from a standing height?" As I continue to argue my case, Mrs Konigsberg enters the room and I invite her to sit down.

"You have to understand, her liver enzymes are elevated and I don't have any of her recent tests. I need to rule out liver damage," I reply, raise my voice a little and startling Mrs Konigsberg. The conversation goes on for a few more minutes while the radiologist persists and I too refuse to back down. We surgeons know how grueling a radiologist's night shift can be, spent mostly in front of a screen deciphering complicated imaging tests with heavy eyelids. However, sometimes we have no choice. In the small hours of the night, we ourselves can become small, and as Samuel Shem describes in his satirical book *The House of God,* doctors are eager to pass the responsibility for their patients onto someone else and go to sleep.

In the end the radiologist gives up his fight. He knows it's a losing battle, that if he refuses I will call Johnny and take our dispute to the next level. Mrs Konigsberg doesn't really want to do an abdominal CT scan, and her son is nervously pacing the ER after ordering a taxi home and assuring me, in a slightly aggressive tone, that he will take care of his mother who he thinks has unnecessarily waited for me in the ER. But I quietly fill out the CT form and go with Mrs Konigsberg to have her scan.

I knock on the door of the radiologist's room and he wearily lets me in, curses and sits back in his chair. Despite his Jekyll and Hyde character, he's an excellent resident and I like him. I notice a bag of gummy snakes on the table and take one, without asking permission, and we proceed to examine the CT on the screen.

"Well, she's got a lacerated liver, looks like a grade III laceration," I mumble, my mouth full of gummy snakes. The radiologist looks a little disgruntled that I was right and he was wrong, and I know I'm rubbing salt in the wound, but I really don't mean to. I feel a sense of satisfaction that I insisted on the CT, even though it means that Mrs

Konigsberg will have to be hospitalized and fully monitored, most likely in the trauma unit.

"Here, take another gummy snake and get out of here," the radiologist retorts, handing me the bag. "I don't want to see you again until morning." He opens the door for me, and despite his irritation, his eyes are smiling and I know he thinks of me differently now, and that next time *if there is any doubt, there will be no doubt.*

I sit with Mrs Konigsberg and her son and explain that in light of the results she will have to be hospitalized for observation for at least for two days.

"In most cases a lacerated liver resolves itself without the need for intervention," I explain. "We just need to see that your blood tests are good and that there is no ongoing bleeding." Mrs Konigsberg and her son are a little surprised, having not expect this scenario, especially from such a minor fall.

"I want to thank you, doctor for insisting on the CT," says the son, a little embarrassed. "May God bless you," he adds, and I smile at them. Mrs Konigsberg looks scared and worried but I know she'll be fine. I leave the ER, hoping not to return for the night, and walk briskly to the ward. It's time to sleep.

4 a.m.

At this hour of the morning the work can be a little erratic. There are usually a few people in the ER who were involved in a car accident or have abdominal pain and are waiting for a surgeon. But for the most part it's quiet, and to an outside observer the ER looks like a dormant volcano, waiting to erupt again. The head nurse rests her head on the counter, taking advantage of a moment's respite. Sleepy interns divide the night between them and look for a place to sleep. The orderlies sit in the staff room glaring at the TV in between transporting patients to various locations. Miraculously tonight most of the patients on the ward in serious condition are asleep.

I sluggishly walk through the dark corridors of the department, looking for a room to lay my head. I know it will be a disturbed sleep, interrupted by at least one phone call from the ER along the lines of: *Is this the on-call surgeon? There's a patient here who's been waiting two hours for an examination,* or *There's a patient here with chest pains and bothering hemorrhoids.* I have no patience at this hour, certainly not for minor cases. I am completely devoid of energy.

It's 4:15 a.m. and I finally find a bed to rest on when Shpet calls me and tells me in a sleepy voice to go see Aaron, there is now more blood in his drains. I had just taken off my shoes, my body screaming with exhaustion, so much so that it takes me a moment to remember who Aaron is and why he has drains.

I curse aloud, put my shoes back on and go to Aaron's room. His wife is standing next to the bed while Ahmed the intern tries to take a blood sample. I glance at Aaron; he's breathing heavily, his abdomen is swollen, his blood pressure is dropping, there is blood in his drains and he's semi-conscious. At this stage I can't sufficiently piece it all together into a clear picture, but I vaguely understand that Aaron has massive intra-abdominal bleeding. I try to inject a needle to take blood, but like Ahmed, I fail, unable to feel any veins due to low blood pressure. Aaron is in hemodynamic shock. I call Shpet,

120

tell him to come quickly. Shpet arrives and tells me to try to inject a needle again, but I am hesitant. I feel that Aaron is slipping through our fingers and that any minute now he will leave this world for a better place.

I tell Shpet that we need emergency blood transfusions—there is no time to wait for the blood bank to prepare Aaron's own match for transfusion, a procedure that usually takes at least an hour—and that we must insert a central line to avoid failed attempts at inserting a peripheral line. Shpet understands the gravity of the situation.

I send Ahmed to the ER for two emergency blood transfusions, type O negative, and in the meantime Shpet inserts a central line into the groin. Aaron is unresponsive by now, his grey face covered in cold sweat. We are running out of time.

After administering the transfusions, we need to rush Aaron to the angiography unit where the interventional radiologist will stop the bleeding. Shpet calls the on-call interventional radiologist, Gil, and explains Aaron's situation in a few words—*a total gastrectomy a week ago, pancreatic leak, blood in drains, hemodynamically unstable*—enough for Gil to go into emergency mode along with us and get to the hospital immediately. It's clear to us by now what has happened: Pancreatic juice that leaked into the abdomen is corroding the sheath of blood vessels in the abdomen, causing the start of acute bleeding into the abdominal cavity. Ahmed returns with the blood transfusions, panting, drops of sweat falling from his forehead. The blood transfusions are still cool but there is no time to warm them up and we hastily connect them to the central line.

We stabilize Aaron's blood pressure and quickly run with him to the angiography unit, leaving his wife behind in the ward, tearful and shocked. I don't have the privilege to look her in the eye and tell her that everything will be fine. These are seconds of life that are running out. At the angiography clinic our friends from interventional radiology come into the picture. Gil, a skilled and talented doctor, has arrived in his pajamas and quickly change into his uniform. Shpet and I lay Aaron down on the treatment bed and clear the area for Gil and his team. Gil rushes into action, administers a local anesthetic within seconds, then pierces Aaron's groin to reveal acute, massive bleeding in the

121

abdominal cavity, originating from intra-abdominal blood vessels. Shpet and I sprawl in the two chairs outside the angiography clinic while Gil stops the bleeding with an emergency catheterization. I fall asleep for a second, a sudden sleep that comes after many hours on my feet. With my head resting on my shoulder, my legs outstretched, I allow myself to relax while Aaron is in someone else's hands. I still have a sweet taste in my mouth of gummy snakes that I ate earlier and my adrenaline rush begins to subside. Gil finishes treating Aaron at around 5 a.m. and we take him back to the ward. Aaron is now completely stable and his wife's tears of pain are replaced by tears of unadulterated joy.

It took several weeks after the incident with Aaron before I able to look back at the dramatic events of that night and fully comprehend how close we were to losing him.

In general, most of our day-to-day work consists of ordinary, simple cases: opening an abscess, sewing up wounds and incisions, receiving patients at the clinic, sitting in morning meetings, attending morning rounds. Ward and ER shifts are taken up with a variety of ordinary tasks, like in every profession.

A shorter part of our work day is dedicated to the important task of diagnosing patients: identifying and treating gall bladder or pancreatic infections; identifying appendicitis, an incarcerated hernia or a cancerous tumor and proceeding with surgery. However, every now and then, a real and unexpected drama occurs, with no warning and without knowing where or when it's going to catch us. And it is these dramas that turn the whole business of being a doctor into something that resonates with us—not for hours or days, but for many years.

I still have about an hour to sleep before Puta and Imrish arrive and the morning will begin, as it does every day, shining upon us. I lie on the bed with its now rumpled sheets that I had neatly tidied before the incident with Aaron. Remnants of adrenaline course through my body not letting me relax, and the drama, now behind me, runs through my head in a blur of flickering images. My phone beeps—the last thing I need right now—and I wonder who could be texting me at this hour. It's Gadi: *Hey, Yaeli, are you awake? Nitzan got up in the night with a 39 fever. I have a meeting first thing in the morning that I have to attend. Any chance you can get home early?* I close my eyes for a second and think. I've put out several fires during this shift, now it's time to put out my personal fires. *I'll try and make it home for 8, I'll see what I can arrange*, I text him back, then put my phone aside and close my eyes again.

5 a.m.

It's still a little dark outside but the first rays of sunlight illuminate the corner of the room. I hear a distant hum in my head and feel the last bit of adrenaline drain from my body, leaving me exhausted. For a brief moment I think how lucky it is that Nitzan has a fever and I get to go home earlier, but quickly dismiss this unmotherly thought—God forgive me! I hope Puta won't be angry that I plan to miss this morning's round, especially since we've been understaffed lately. Thankfully today is a clinic day with no elective surgeries. Gadi texts me again: *Do you think she needs antibiotics?*

I'm not only a mother, I'm also my family's doctor, shouldering my dad's medical questions and my mom's worries. Sometimes when my sister calls me, I answer her in a panic, anxious that something terrible may have happened, and it takes me a few seconds to calm myself. I have stitched up Gadi's father in the ER, interpreted his mother's ECGs, and I always help the family in whatever way I can, whether it's prescribing medications, dressing wounds or offering advice. But I'm not only my family's doctor, I'm also the apartment building's doctor, treating seizures and minor falls and always giving medical advice to neighbors who ask for it. I'm also the doctor in Nitzan's class and Tamar's class, and because I am always available for others, I often forget to be my own doctor. Like the time I stood for hours in surgery with a cold and a stubborn runny nose, having no choice but to ride it out. And like the time I had a terrible migraine on a weekend shift and had to remind myself to take a pill every three hours to relieve the dizziness and throbbing pain in my temples.

And when my two worlds—me the doctor and me the person—collide, it's hard to separate them, and everything gets mixed up, like in a real collision: the anxiety with the complacency; the fact that I know with the fact that I don't know everything; and above all, the fact that it's so close to me, that it's someone from my family, that it's now like me and myself. And who can lift me out from the collision of these two worlds? A few months ago, I experienced such a collision and the memory of it is still fresh and deep.

It was a Sunday, about 10 p.m. and I was on duty in the ER with Johnny and Gravitz, another senior resident. It was relatively quiet when out of the blue my sister Adi called me. Five days earlier she had given birth to her first child.

"I've started bleeding," she said. "I think some stitches have opened, what should I do?"

Adi is my only sister, born after many years of waiting for a sibling, and we are very close; always there for each in good times and in bad. I wasn't sure what to tell her about the bleeding. She had a newborn at home and a husband who could barely come to grips with the fact that he was a father, and I felt it might be difficult for her to come to the ER. Yet something in her voice told me that it was not just a few open stitches, but something more serious, so, I advised her to come and find out what was wrong. I anxiously waited for her and meanwhile examined a patient who had fallen and had rib pain. Adi called me again and spoke quickly, her voice weak.

"Yael, I'm here in the parking lot near the ER. I can't get out of the car, I'm constantly bleeding." I muttered a few sentences to the patient I was examining, sent him for a chest x-ray and ran to the parking lot, grabbing a wheelchair on the way. I helped my pale-faced sister out of the car and called Johnny and Gravitz.

"Come quick, my sister has postpartum bleeding, Meet me in the shock room." Johnny and Gravitz showed up immediately, together with the nurse. We inserted two large intravenous lines into my sister's arm, took blood samples for crossmatching and ordered doses of blood to be on the safe side. I arranged for the orderly to transport me and my sister to the gynecology building and I also spoke with the on-call gynecologist. By this time, my sister was still bleeding and we had already changed her bandages twice. In the transport vehicle she lay on a bed and I stood next to her, regulating my breathing and thinking. I held the handgrip above my head as the vehicle made twists and turns around the hospital and I tried to put a smile on my sister's face. And then the collision came, the anxiety, made worse by the fact that I had left the ER—which could erupt at any minute— in the middle of my shift. Johnny and Gravitz covered for me, running between patients. They texted me that everything was under control and I should stay with my sister.

When we finally arrived at the gynecology building, a nice nurse told him about my sister's bleeding, but he dismissed my concerns and wasn't very reassuring.

"There are much more urgent cases here," he said. "It sounds to me like everything will be fine, but it will be a while before I can see your sister." In medical jargon we call this personnel-itis—a medical complication that could have been avoided that occurs in a patient who is a member or relative of the hospital staff. People always think it's beneficial to have connections with or be related to medical professionals. But this is actually a misconception, because in most cases this connection breeds two evils: the first is overtreatment, such as when a big-name specialist comes to check on a patient who is a member of the hospital staff and is overconfident, smug, and lacks the creativity and curiosity that a young resident may possess; and undertreatment, the tendency of a doctor to be over-reassuring, neglectful, complacent. Because how is it possible that Dreznik's sister's condition is life-threatening?

I tried calling my parents. It was already midnight and my sister was still bleeding. The doctors injected her with something that shrinks the uterus and which I learned about in gynecology rotation, but I couldn't remember what it was called and how effective it was. And why on earth hadn't the bleeding stopped and why did so many blood clots show up on my sister's ultrasound ? I know what I saw in the ultrasound images, but I bought into the reassuring words of the gynecologist, his confidence that the situation was under control, and that in a short time the bleeding would stop. At 3 a.m. I tried calling my parents again, but there was no answer. Thank God Johnny and Gravitz were covering for me because there was no way I was going to leave my sister.

I didn't notice how pale my sister looked, probably because of the strong neon lighting and the fact that we both tried to deal with the situation by telling our own private jokes. But when she was taken for another examination in the early morning and her blood pressure had dropped and her hemoglobin was below 10 gm/dL, I realized she was in hemodynamic shock. The problem is that I realized this a little late because I had fallen into the trap of the gynecologist's complacency, the sense that everything will be okay because Adi is my sister. But luckily, I came to my senses just in time, just as my father called, his concern reverberating through my phone speaker.

"Yael, were you looking for us? Is everything alright?" I gathered myself together. I was the family doctor now, not a hysterical sister. "Yes, don't worry, Adi is here at the hospital, she was bleeding a little. She's being treated but I need you to come. Everything is fine."

After a couple of hours, my sister was finally stabilized. And although today we can look back and laugh a little about the bloodbath, it is always there—that inevitable collision between the doctor, the wife, the mother, the daughter and the sister that I am.

I glare at the shards of light breaking through the window shutters in the on-call room and return to my dual role of mother and doctor, wondering how to answer Gadi.

I don't think Nitzani needs antibiotics, I text him. *I'll take care of her when I get home. It sounds like a virus.* I don't know what a virus sounds like and I don't know if I'm right. I used my mother's intuition mixed together with a bit of doctor's insight and a lot of fatigue. It's the best I can do at 5:50 a.m. The morning round is about to begin.

6 a.m.

The transition from night shift to morning always follows the same pattern: I wake up cold and dizzy after very little sleep and wash my face and brush my teeth which fails to refreshen me. And yet, I feel a sense of elation that my shift is finally over, especially after a night of saving lives, making the right decisions and successful surgeries. It's heartwarming to go home with a gift or a letter of appreciation from a patient's family and to pass the baton with a feeling of accomplishment. Fortunately, our shift hours are fairly reasonable nowadays, unlike the past when residents had to work another whole day after a 26-hour shift; simply inhumane. Not long before our shifts were reduced to a maximum of 26 hours, we would work about 30-hour shifts and go home at around 1 p.m., exhausted in a way I can't describe in words. About a year ago I stayed at the hospital until 5 p.m. after a night shift, but that's because I couldn't leave earlier; my conscience wouldn't let me. I had been on my way out of the hospital when Nitzan's nanny, Simcha, had called me crying. "It's Jacob my husband," she said, "he's not well."

I got to know Jacob while Simcha was Nitzan's nanny. A quiet, introverted man, a devoted husband, a good and beloved father. He and Simcha lived close to us. He was 70 years old, a relatively healthy person with no underlying illnesses. It turned out that for some time he had been suffering from abdominal pain that got worse and was accompanied by vomiting. Simcha took him to the ER. Until then they only knew me as Yael, Nitzan's mother, but after treating Jacob in the ER they got to know Yael the surgeon. Jacob's abdominal x-ray was abnormal, there were distended bowel loops and signs of intestinal obstruction. I took him for an abdominal CT scan and a tumor was detected in the small intestine. I and another senior doctor operated on him and found an adenocarcinoma, an obstructing tumor in the small intestine. Within a few days Jacob went home and began biological therapy, but his condition did not really improve.

Tumors of this type in the small intestine, unlike the large intestine, are less good in terms of prognosis, progression and treatment.

So, when Simcha called me at work in tears, I figured that the disease had progressed. We hospitalized Jacob and put him on parenteral nutrition. An additional CT scan revealed extensive progression of the disease. The entire abdominal cavity was filled with lumps, a real catastrophe, especially since the disease was inoperable. Jacob received a lot of morphine but he was in terrible pain due to bowel obstruction. In our staff meeting with the boss and Jacob's oncologist it was decided to operate to try to resolve the obstruction. The decision was made during my shift, and it was clear to me, and also to Simcha and Jacob, that I would stay with them and attend the surgery However, the surgery was postponed until noon the following day, and although my shift had ended by then, I stayed behind.

At noon I entered the OR exhausted and waited for the surgery to begin. Only at 2:30 p.m. did we finally wheel Jacob into the OR. I saw Simcha and I felt that it calmed her knowing I was there. Even though I had only been a resident for a year and didn't yet know the ins and outs of Jacob's surgery, I did know that healing is a combination of body and soul, and that right now I was Simcha and Jacobs soul. At 3 p.m., after tedious preparations, I helped the attending carefully open Jacob's abdomen and found many lumps of tumor and an enlarged, swollen intestine. The prognosis was clear and the purpose of the surgery was to ease Jacobs's pain and to give him a few more months of life without suffering. I had not slept for over thirty hours, my muscles ached and exhaustion seeped into every pore of my body, but I fought it off and mustered up whatever energy I had left to get through the surgery. Jacob's bowel was so friable and enlarged, it perforated during surgery and feces filled the abdominal cavity. The attending and I realized that there wasn't much we could do without causing more damage except to take out a stoma where the bowel was perforated to help clear the obstruction and then close the abdomen. It was one of those horrible moments when, weak in the knees, you explain to the family that it was difficult, that you tried all you could, the situation is not good but you hope he will recover. But my eyes offer no glimmer of hope.

After Jacob's surgery, my long and debilitating shift was finally over, and on the way home it's a miracle I didn't fall asleep at the wheel. I arrived home at 5:30 pm, picked up Nitzan, and took her to her school for the "Borrow a Book" project. I didn't even have time to change out of my uniform I had been wearing since the previous before. The school secretary informed me that I was supposed to fill out some form and bring a check, which I had forgotten to bring, and without it we couldn't participate in the project. At that moment, with my abysmal fatigue, I broke down in tears in front of the secretary, my daughter and several other startled mothers. "Come on," I said to Nitzan, who didn't understand what had happened to me and why my eyes were swollen from crying. "I'll buy you books for school without this project." Nitzan was overjoyed and we walked hand in hand to the car, she with thoughts of new books, and I with Jacob in my heart.

I have worked several long, exhausting shifts like this one, which ended long after my feet could carry me, and I always ask myself, as do most doctors, why we are expected to function like this and how could our overloaded schedule be managed differently. Yet I know that even if we were to work less hours, fatigue would probably always remain an inherent part of our work.

It's 5:55 a.m. and I hear Puta's footsteps in the long corridor of the ward which is still dark. We residents know each other's footsteps, each other's small gestures, tone of voice and silent looks in morning meetings when the senior physicians argue with each other or criticize us. Sometimes I see the other residents on weekends and holidays more than I see my own family. And the power of this togetherness, woven into the fabric of our work, is what gets us through our residency and keeps us sane.

" I see you slept well last night, Dreznik," Puta remarks. Sometimes I don't know if he is being serious or not. He turns on the laptop and calls to Ahmed the intern— who, like me, is also clearly exhausted from lack of sleep—to come to the nurses' station.

"It was hell," I say to Puta, adding details about Aaron and his bleeding and about Weitzner, who is now dying in recovery unit. Even Puta, with all his cynicism and something to say about everything, looks at me in silence for a few seconds. "Wow, madness," he says under his breath and turns to the laptop to looks at Aaron's vitals and Weitzner 's surgery report. Imrish arrives and tosses back his forelock. It's 6.10 a.m. and Puta reprimands him for being late. "We have a guy with jaundice on the ward. Aviad," I continue to update. "I hope it's just a stone in the bile ducts. He needs to go for an ultrasound as soon as the institute opens. And I have to go home in an hour, my little one is sick and there's no one to replace me." Imrish and Puta are understanding, even if it means they will have to work harder than usual today. Imrish winks at me and brings me a piece of chocolate from the nurses' station, which he calls the 'chocolate for champions' who survived the night shift, and if I had been staying for the break on the ramp, he would have bought me 'coffee for champions'. Puta and Imrish wheel the laptop to one of the rooms and Ahmed and I, together with two other interns, follow them. The morning round has begun.

7 a.m.

Mom, dad wants to know if you'll be home by 8, Tamar texts me. I smile at the phone. *Yes, I'll make it home by then,* I text her back.

Okay mom, I love you, and don't worry about Nitzan, she's here next to me taking her temperature. Oh and please don't forget to buy me an erasable pen for school, followed by a smiley and a small red heart. It's always non-stop texting with Tamar, which makes me laugh every time. I place the phone in my pocket and leave the main building.

It's a few minutes' walk to the pediatric building. It's already 7:15 a.m. and I only have a few minutes before running home to release Gadi.

"Where's the baby who underwent surgery for intussusception? Yuval something..." I ask at the nurses' station, trying to remember his last name. "Yes, Yuval Rabinovitch, room 6," the head nurse replies, and I walk quickly to the room. Yuval is sleeping calmy with a pacifier in his mouth, his parents next to him. They immediately recognize me.

"Doctor Yael!" the mother says, excited to see me. We only met yesterday for the first time, a short while before I was inside her son's body, and here we are again a day after the surgery.

"How is the little one feeling?" I ask with a broad smile, seeing Dr Shenhav out of the corner of my eye preparing for his morning round.

"He's doing great, the mother replies. "He's eaten a little, pooped..." The father stands next to me, looking at his wife, then they both smile at me, a beautiful smile that no words can describe. I don't want to wake Yuval from his peaceful sleep. Soon doctor Shenhav will examine him, see that everything is fine and discharge him.

I go to say hello to Dr Shenhav, we are happy to see each other.

"When are you coming to us for pediatric surgery residency?" he asks with a questioning smile, and I know in my heart that this day will come; there's something about children that beats it all.

Before I stopped by baby Yuval, I did two more things that I had promised myself to do. The first was to check in on Shani with the breast tumor. It's a rule I've never broken: to check in on patients the morning after I've operated on them, no matter whether the surgery was big or small. Shani was already walking around the ward, calm and in less pain. I prepared a discharge letter for her, wished her and her husband good health, and hoped that the lymph node we removed would be tumor-free and that everything would be fine. The second thing I did was to visit Mr Weitzner in recovery, along with Johnny and Shpet. He was sedated and ventilated and his blood pressure was very low. Shpet hugged his children who sat sad-eyed next to him; he had nothing more to offer. It was agreed with the recovery unit that Mr Weitzner would come to our ward for a morphine drip, our euphemism for a painless death. We talked to the family some more and on the way out of the recovery room Johnny tossed a few swear words in the air. I parted from Shpet and Johnny and they went to the ramp together for some oxygen before their day began.

On my way to the pediatric building, I meet Aviad and Dana who are heading to the ultrasound unit, and my heart goes out to them. "What about our coffee and cigarette?" Dana asks me. "You promised me!" I smile back at her, praying that Aviad's examination goes well.

I look for my car in the parking lot. I always try to park it in the same spot so as not to forget where it is, which has happened a number of times. There are countless stories of residents who after a night shift, spend an hour or more looking for their car, or try to open it with a credit card instead of keys, or once they are home suddenly fall asleep while talking to a family member. The sun blinds me and I drag my weary feet a few more steps, in anticipation of sleep. Puta informs us on the residents' Whatsapp group that Aharon is in stable condition, but that Shpet and Dr Vasser will probably perform surgery on him this morning to remove the blood clots that have accumulated in his abdomen. I think of how exhausted Shpet must be after a long and difficult night. I feel a little guilty for leaving him and the others to manage the ward alone, but I am grateful to be going home.

In the car I listen to Bob Dylan's "One More Cup of Coffee" at high volume, a song that always reminds me of the beginning of residency. I nervously approach the traffic light at the hospital exit, where on more than one occasion I have closed my dreary eyes for a second, only to be woken up and startled by the hooting of cars behind me. But at that moment Puta calls me, heightening my senses. I hope everything is okay and that I didn't mess up during the night.

"Dreznik, I just want to let you know," he says in his friendly, laconic manner. "Aviad with the jaundice who you hospitalized? Don't ask. He has a huge tumor in the head of the pancreas. Metastases in the liver. God forgive you for leaving me to deal with this alone." We exchange a few more words and I hang up with a choking feeling in my throat, unable to breath.

At exactly 8 a.m. Gadi greets me at the door. There's a sweet smell of home, some clothes and toys lie scattered on the floor. Nitzan is lying on the couch as she does when she is sick, watching TV, covered with a blanket from her room. I am struck by the seeming incongruence between this reality and my reality of the past twenty-six hours. How it is that these two realities coexist?

"Was it a hard shift?" Gadi asks me, just before he leaves for work. He knows me, he can tell when I'm suffocating, when I don't have the words to describe what I've been through.

I join Nitzan on the couch and she wraps me in her warm little arms, her eyes a little glassy from the fever, but she seems fine to me. I hug her tightly, inhaling her good, innocent smell, and tears flow from my eyes involuntarily.

"Mom had a difficult shift," I tell her, and she looks at me.

"Mom, tomorrow will be a good day!" she replies. Tomorrow is Tuesday and on Tuesdays we learn in groups a school. I love Tuesdays. You too will have a good day tomorrow," she adds. I marvel at her maturity and ability to contain me, then close my eyes. Darkness.

Epilogue

Aviad, who came to the ER with obstructive jaundice, was diagnosed with an advanced stage of pancreatic cancer. He underwent chemotherapy but died a number of months later in the oncology department at the age of forty-five.

Aharon, who had massive bleeding after a total gastrectomy, was hospitalized for an extended period in intensive care but was present at the birth of his first granddaughter. He was discharged home but died a year and a half later due to the progression of the disease and additional metastases.

Osnat, who was diagnosed with diffuse carcinoma of unknown origin, was hospitalized and began chemotherapy. She died a few months after the diagnosis.

Shani, who underwent a lumpectomy to remove a malignant breast tumor, did follow-up at a breast clinic with no evidence of recurrence of the disease. The lymph node was found to be tumor-free and the removed tumor margins were found to be clean.

Mrs Konigsberg, who was diagnosed with liver hematoma as the result of a fall, was hospitalized for three days' observation in the trauma unit and was discharged home in good general condition.

Mr Sa'adi, who suffered from kidney failure and bleeding hemorrhoids received blood transfusions through a central line. He subsequently underwent a hemorrhoidectomy and was discharged home.

Baby Yuval, who underwent surgery for intussusception, came to the clinic for a check-up a week after surgery with a normal-looking scar and in excellent general condition.

Ten Rules of General Surgery

1. Eat when you can, sleep when you can, and don't mess with the pancreas.

2. It's not ER, it's PR.

3. All bleeding eventually stops.

4. The surgical resident is like a mushroom: kept in the dark, fed shit, and expected to grow.

5. Surgery is not an art: it's a personality disorder.

6. Never let the sun set on bowel obstruction.

7. There is an inverse relationship between the surgeon's ability and the frequency he asks for more muscle relaxants.

8. It's never a gynecological problem according to the gynecologist.

9. Surgery is not easy. To pee in the bath is.

10. What is the difference between a surgeon and God? God knows he is not a surgeon.

Acknowledgements

This was my first shift. I sat on the couch in the living room with my laptop and in what was to become a regular ritual, I poured out my heart about all I had been through in the longest day of my like. I wrote about the fear of the unknown, the fatigue due to endless hours of work, coping with death, a serious illness and with families who are thrown into an unfamiliar and threatening world. I wrote about myself in all this chaos, without pausing to breathe.

A few years have passed since then, and the year of the coronavirus pandemic and its forced silence motivated me to reexamine my collection of hospital stories that remained in the drawer, and the idea arose to turn them into a book. The words simply wrote themselves, accurately describing events that took place, surgeries that were performed, the tears cried, and the patients who, to this day, melt my heart.

I also wish to express my deepest thanks to my colleagues in the medical profession, the residents, specialists, nurses and students, who are forever in my thoughts and who accompany me in the most difficult moments, unmatched by any other profession and who will always be like a second family to me.

I am also immensely grateful to my beloved friends who relentlessly support me on the long journey I have chosen, and for reading the initial draft with enthusiasm and love.

I wish to give special thanks to my family, my true driving force and the reason for my life, for their unwavering support without which I would not have realized my dreams, and in particular I thank my two wonderful daughters, Tamar and Nitzan.

Finally, I wish to thank all the patients who made me the doctor I am—from the premature baby who was born weighing half a kilogram and needed emergency surgery, to the 96-year-old man who was rushed to the operating table, and the thousands of beloved patients who etched into my flesh the meaning of giving and who make me want to be a doctor every day.